Erythrocyte

Edited by Anil Tombak

Published in London, United Kingdom

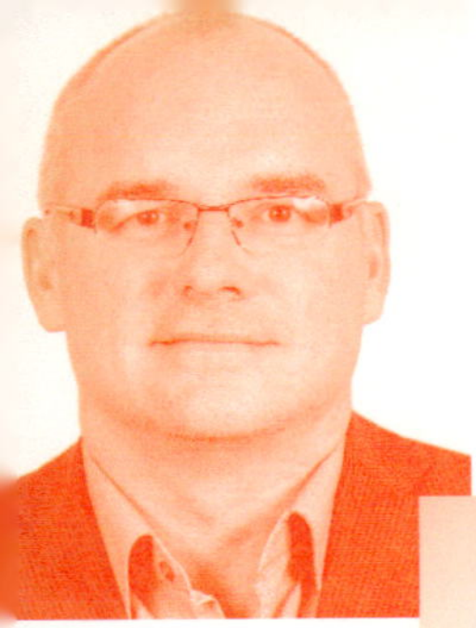

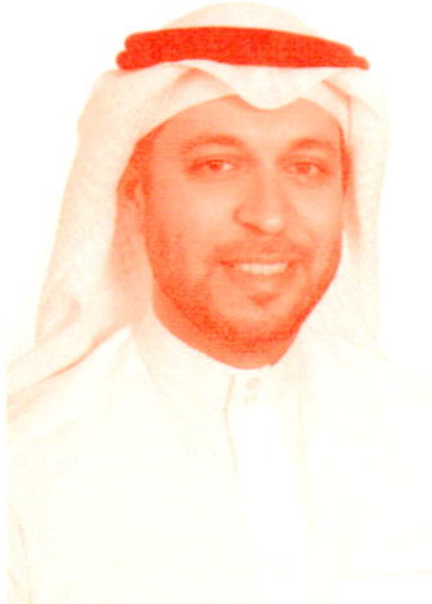

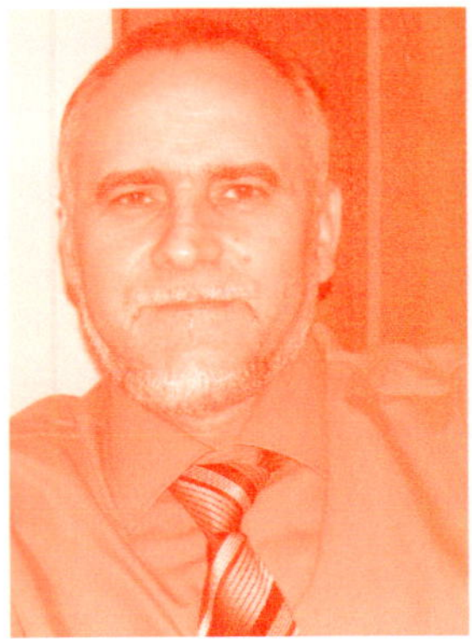

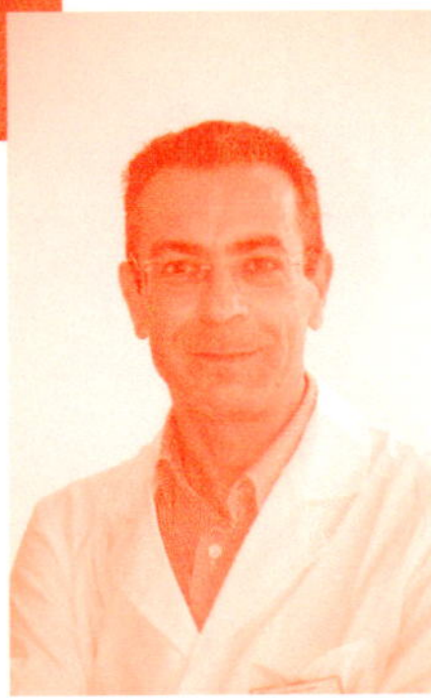

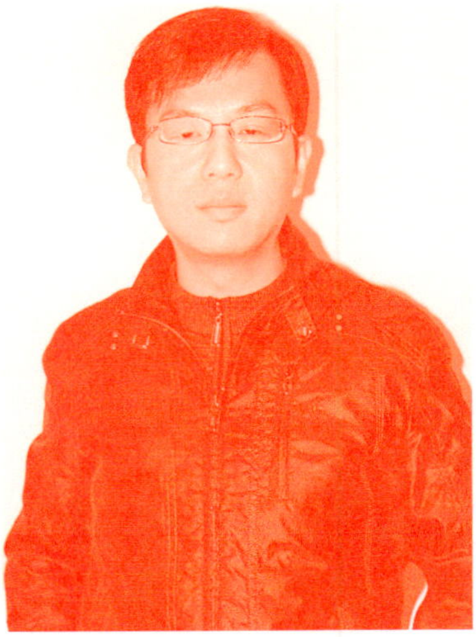

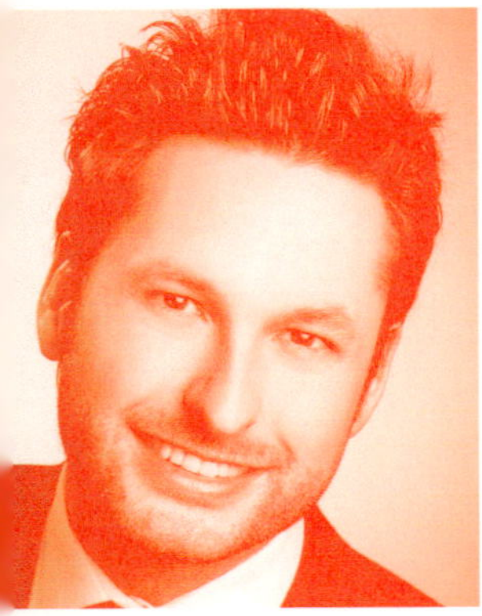

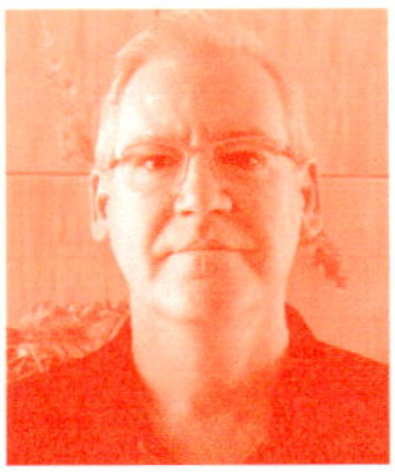

IntechOpen

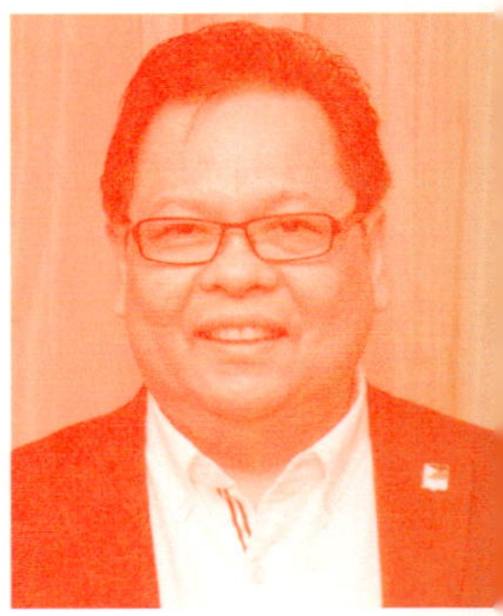

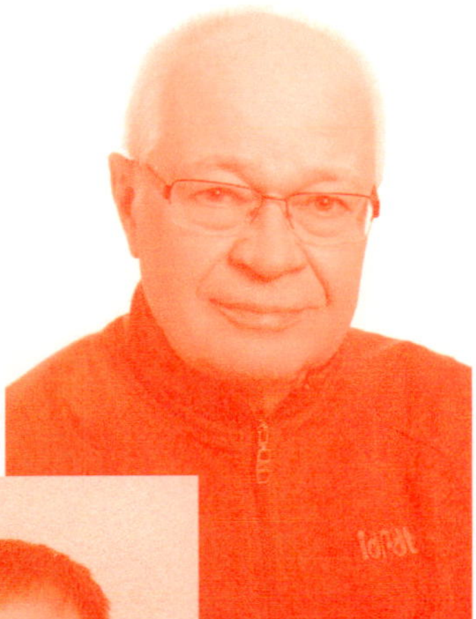

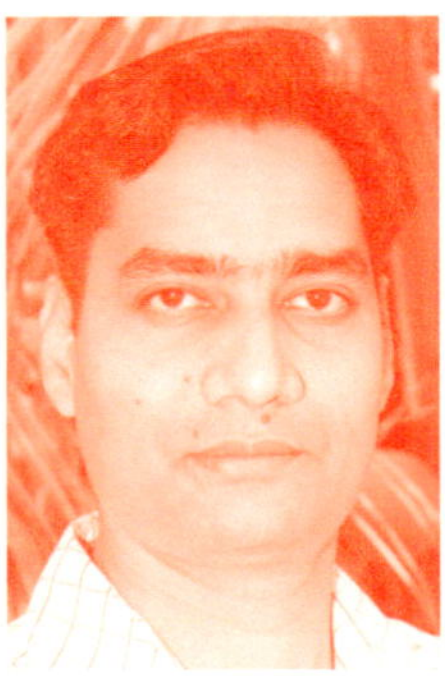

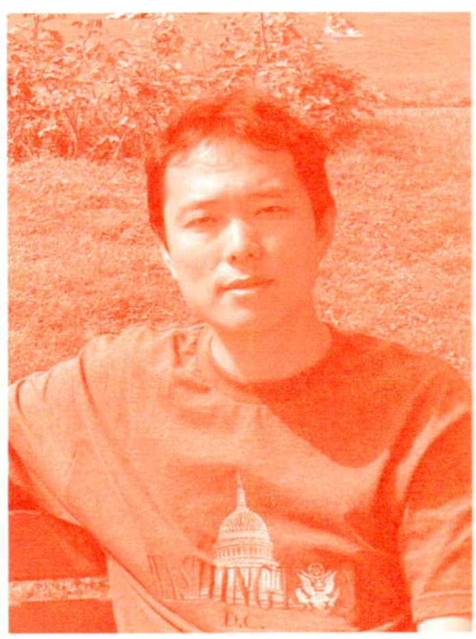

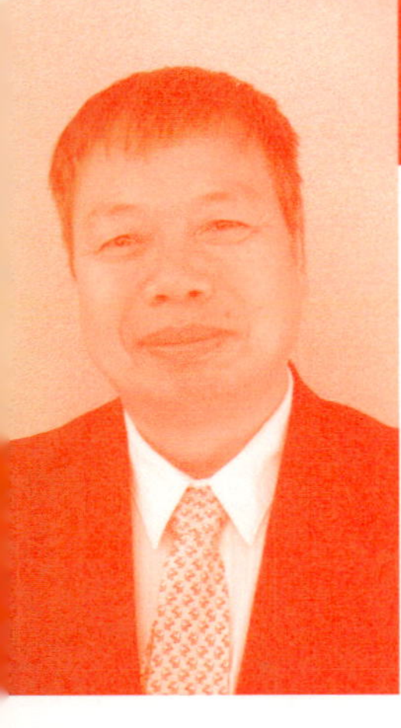

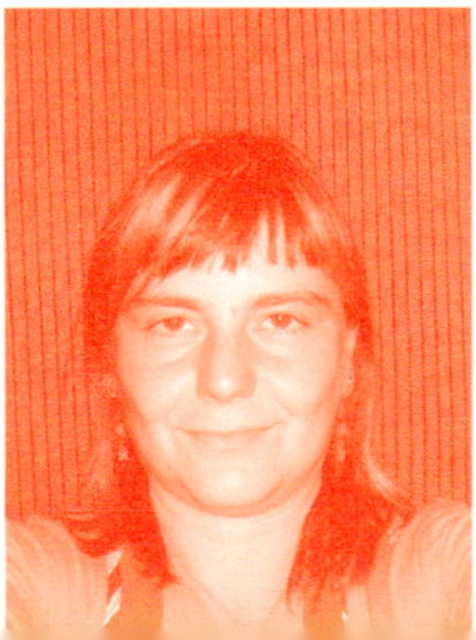

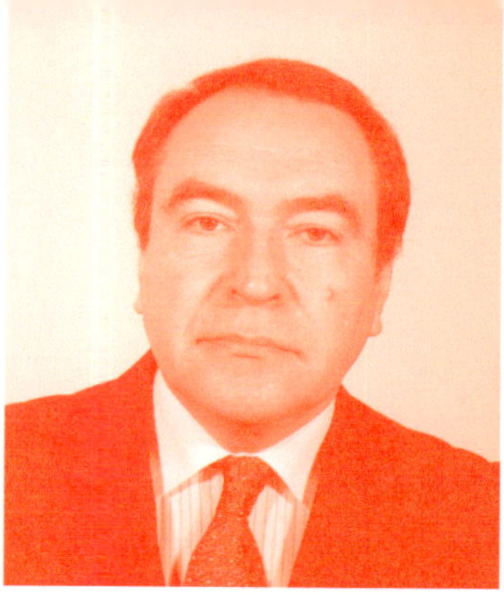
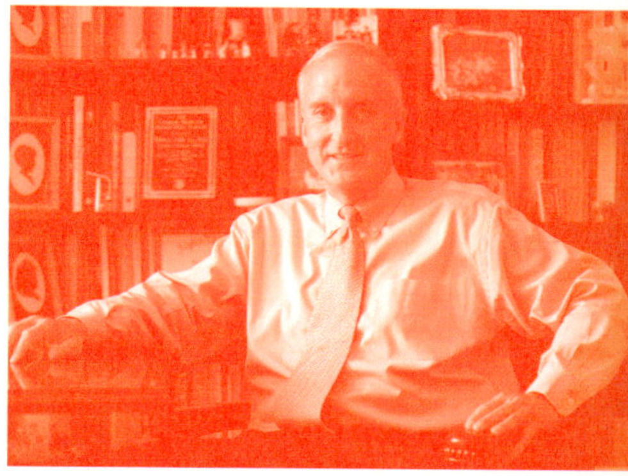
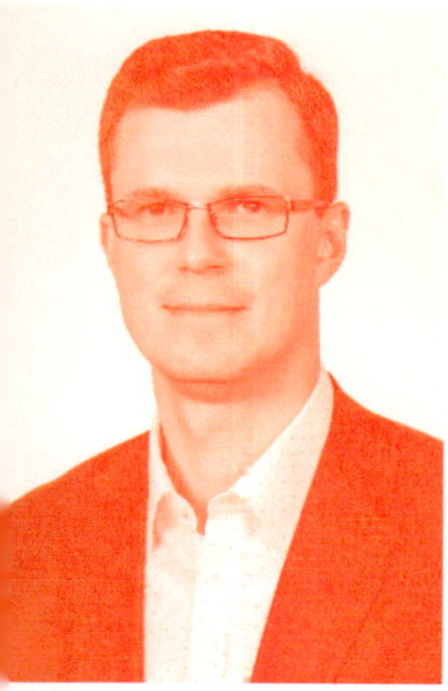
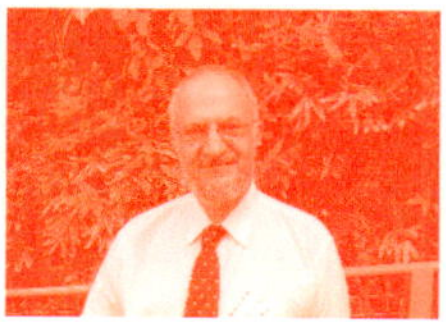
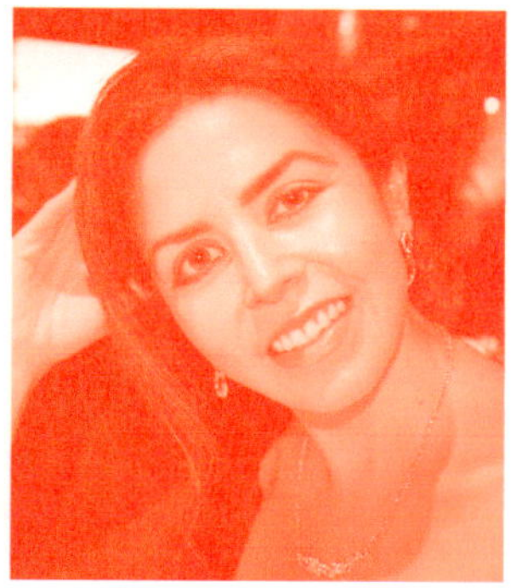

Supporting open minds since 2005

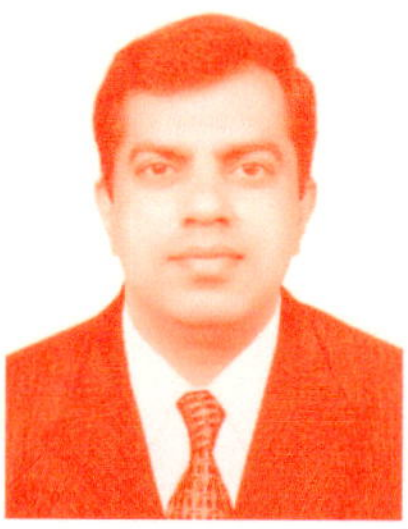
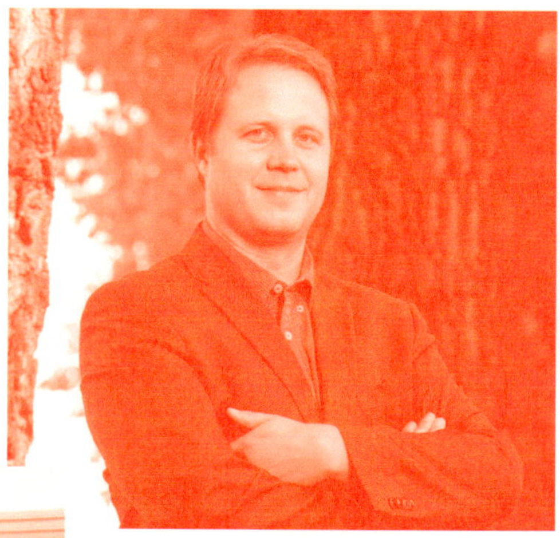
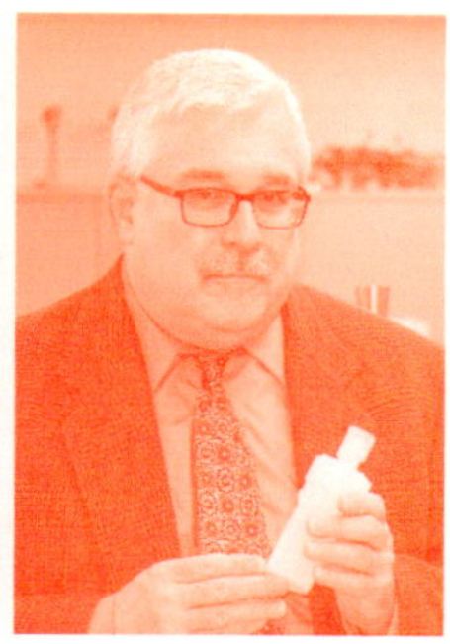
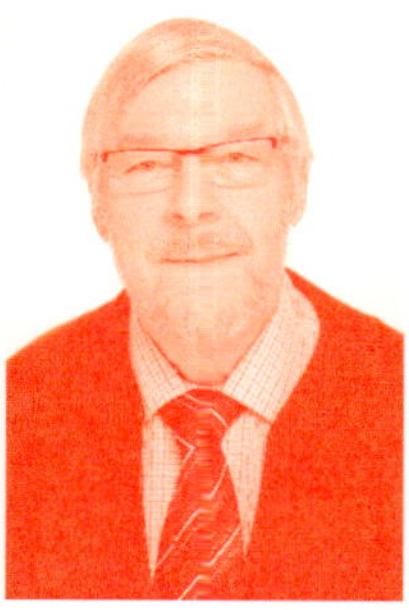
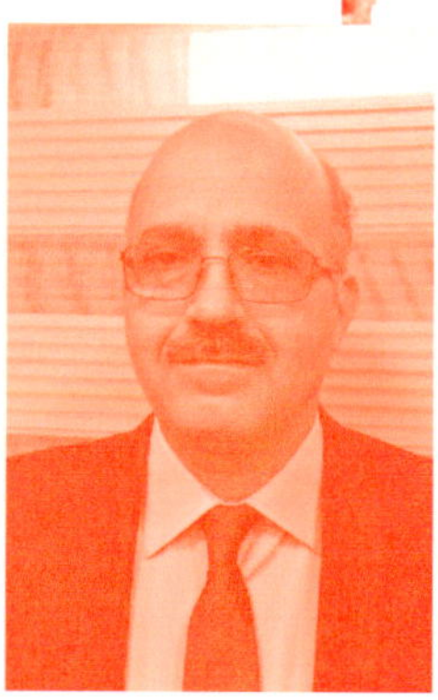
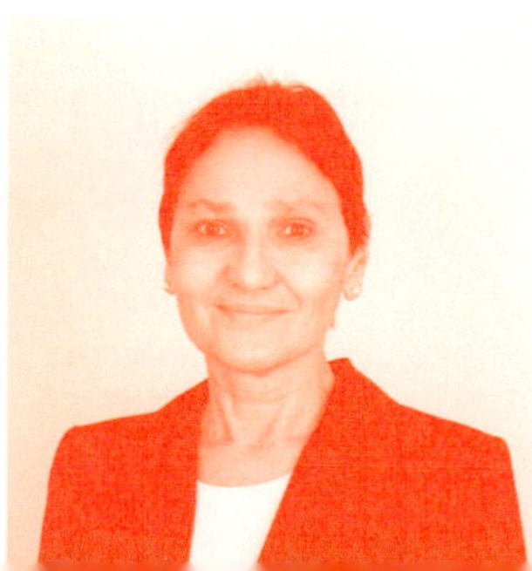
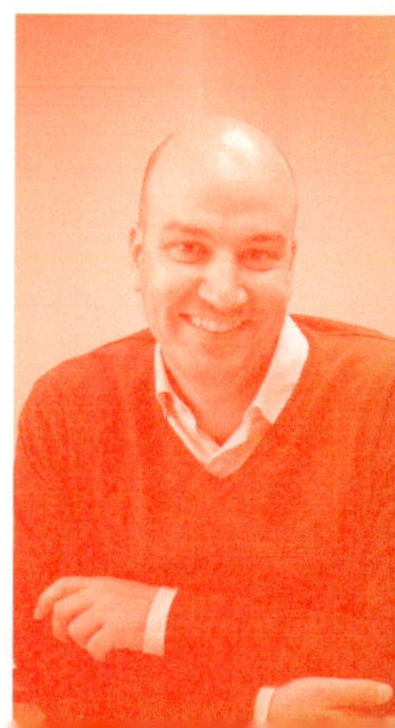

Erythrocyte
http://dx.doi.org/10.5772/intechopen.73981
Edited by Anil Tombak

Contributors
Minh T.N. Le, Daniel Xin Zhang, Theodoros Kiomourtzis, Chun Kuen Lam, Marcy C. Purnell, Risa D. Ramsey, Ingolf Bernhardt, Lars Kaestner, Duc Bach Nguyen, Mauro C. Wesseling, T. Rajini Samuel, Gyudo Lee, Insu Kim, Dae Sung Yoon, Alice Santos Silva, Daniela Melo, Susana Rocha, Susana Coimbra, Eitan Fibach, Mutaz Dana, Ademola Samson Adewoyin, Oluwafemi Adeyemi, Nosimot Omolola Davies, Ann Abiola Ogbenna, Saganuwan Alhaji Saganuwan, Anil Tombak

First published in London, United Kingdom, 2019 by IntechOpen
IntechOpen is the global imprint of INTECHOPEN LIMITED, registered in England and Wales, registration number: 11086078, The Shard, 25th floor, 32 London Bridge Street
London, SE19SG – United Kingdom
Printed in Croatia

British Library Cataloguing-in-Publication Data
A catalogue record for this book is available from the British Library

Additional hard and PDF copies can be obtained from orders@intechopen.com

Erythrocyte
Edited by Anil Tombak
p. cm.
Print ISBN 978-1-78984-209-8
Online ISBN 978-1-78984-210-4
eBook (PDF) ISBN 978-1-78984-693-5

For EU product safety concerns:
IN TECH d.o.o., Prolaz Marije Krucifikse Kozulić 3, 51000 Rijeka, Croatia, info@intechopen.com or visit our website at intechopen.com.

Meet the editor

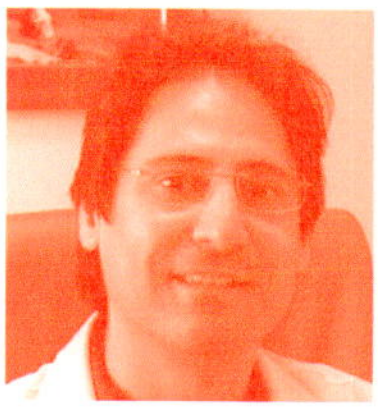

Assoc. Prof. Dr. Anil Tombak, MD, was born on April 25, 1976. He graduated from Gazi Anatolian High School in 1994, and then from Çukurova University Medical Faculty in 2000. Subsequently, he was trained at Mersin University Medical Faculty Internal Medicine Department, and after internal medicine specialization became a fellow of hematology at the same university. He became a hematologist in 2013 while still working at Mersin University Medical Faculty, Department of Internal Medicine—Hematology, Mersin, Turkey. He has performed research in several fields, and has more than 50 publications in (inter)national journals and numerous papers in scientific conferences. He has received several awards and is a member of the Turkish Society of Hematology. Dr. Tombak is married and has two children.

Contents

Preface **XI**

Section 1
Erythrocytes: Physiology and Pathophysiology **1**

Chapter 1 **3**
Introductory Chapter: Erythrocytes - Basis of Life
by Anil Tombak

Chapter 2 **7**
Erythrocyte Morphology and Its Disorders
by Ademola Samson Adewoyin, Oluwafemi Adeyemi, Nosimot Omolola Davies and Ann Abiola Ogbenna

Chapter 3 **17**
Red Blood Cells Actively Contribute to Blood Coagulation and Thrombus Formation
by Ingolf Bernhardt, Mauro C. Wesseling, Duc Bach Nguyen and Lars Kaestner

Chapter 4 **33**
Who Is Balancing: Is It RBC or Acid-Base Status?
by T. Rajini Samuel

Chapter 5 **49**
Red Blood Cells as Redox Modulators in Hemolytic Anemia
by Eitan Fibach and Mutaz Dana

Chapter 6 **65**
Interplay between Erythrocyte Peroxidases and Membrane
by Daniela Melo, Susana Rocha, Susana Coimbra and Alice Santos Silva

Chapter 7 **85**
Effects of Therapeutic and Toxic Agents on Erythrocytes of Different Species of Animals
by Saganuwan Alhaji Saganuwan

Section 2
Future Perspectives 119

Chapter 8 121
The Biology and Therapeutic Applications of Red Blood Cell Extracellular Vesicles
by Daniel Xin Zhang, Theodoros Kiomourtzis, Chun Kuen Lam and Minh T.N. Le

Chapter 9 137
Application of Red Cell Membrane in Nanobiotechnology
by Insu Kim, Gyudo Lee and Dae Sung Yoon

Chapter 10 151
The Influence of the Golden Ratio on the Erythrocyte
by Marcy C. Purnell and Risa D. Ramsey

Preface

Today, information in medical science increases rapidly and with the communication age, accessing information is quite easy. However, with this increasing knowledge, information complexity has emerged. Thus, despite all this increasing knowledge, the interest in and need for basic books has not diminished.

Red blood cells constitute approximately 40% of the total amount of blood and 99% of shaped elements of blood. Their major function is oxygen transportation and this makes erythrocytes "the basis of life." However, as readers will see in this book, erythrocytes have a lot of different, important functions in our body. We have learned a great deal so far, but there is still more to learn about erythrocytes. Erythrocyte evolution continues and this book plans to collect current information related to erythrocytes.

I would like to thank all the authors and IntechOpen in the hope that this book will be a stepping stone for scientists who are rapidly advancing their science journey

Dr. Anil Tombak, MD
Associate Professor
Department of Internal Medicine—Hematology,
Mersin University Medical Faculty, Mersin,
Turkey

Section 1

Erythrocytes: Physiology and Pathophysiology

Chapter 1

Introductory Chapter: Erythrocytes - Basis of Life

Anil Tombak

1. Introduction

Erythrocytes (**Figure 1**) constitute approximately 40% of the total amount of the blood and 99% of shaped elements in the blood. They are biconcave disk-shaped cells with an average diameter of 6.2–8.2 μm, a thickness at the thickest point of 2–2.5 μm, and a minimum thickness in the center of 0.8–1 μm. These dimensions make the red blood cells smaller than most other human cells. One millimeter cube of blood contains 5,100,000–5,800,000 erythrocytes in men and 4,300,000–5,200,000 red blood cells in women. These numbers may vary according to age, gender, and height of place [1].

The red blood cells are produced in the vitellus sac during the first few weeks of the fetus, in the spleen, lymph nodes, and liver in the second trimester, and in the bone marrow in the last month before and after birth. Red blood cells are produced in the bone marrow of all bones up to 5 years of age; after the age of 20, they are produced in the bone marrow of vertebrae, sternum, ribs, and iliac bone. All circulating cells are formed by dividing hemopoietic stem cells in the bone marrow.

The production of red blood cells is controlled by erythropoietin hormone produced by the kidneys (90%) and by the liver (10%). The production of red blood cells begins as immature cells in the bone marrow and they mature approximately 7 days later and are released into the blood stream. Initially, the red blood cells are added to the circulation in the form of reticulocytes and reticulocytes become erythrocytes in circulation within 2 days. Reticulocytes typically contain remnants of organelles. Reticulocytes should comprise approximately 1–2% of the erythrocyte count. When oxygen decreases in tissues, the erythropoietin hormone level rises, and red blood cell production is stimulated; however, after 5 days, the new red blood cells appear in the circulation. Abnormally low or high levels of reticulocytes indicate deviations in the production of these erythrocytes.

Red blood cells lack endoplasmic reticula and do not synthesize proteins. They lack mitochondria as well and rely on anaerobic respiration. However, erythrocytes contain a special protein called hemoglobin, which carries oxygen from the lungs to other parts of the body and carries carbon dioxide into the lungs. No mitochondria mean that erythrocytes do not utilize any of the oxygen they are transporting, so they can deliver it all to the tissues. Approximately 90% of red blood cells are hemoglobin. Erythrocytes allow regulation of acid-base balance through hemoglobin. The hemoglobin level in whole blood is 16 g/dl in men and 14 g/dl in women. In a red blood cell, there is an average of 270–300 million molecules of hemoglobin. Each hemoglobin molecule contains four globin groups, each of which can bind a molecule of oxygen. Total iron in the body is 4–5 g, and 65% of this is found in hemoglobin. Hemoglobin molecule gives the red color to the erythrocytes and to the blood.

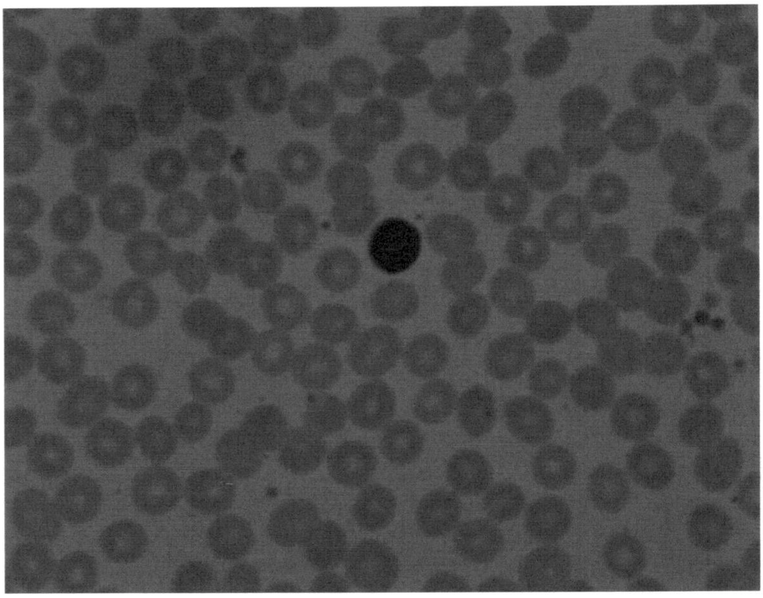

Figure 1.
Light microscopic micrographs of peripheral blood. Normocytic normochromic erythrocytes with central pallor. Central pallor is one-third the size of a red blood cell.

While the major function of red blood cells is hemoglobin-mediated oxygen transport through the body, they also actively participate in both arterial and venous thrombosis, since erythrocytes are the most abundant blood cells, comprising 35–45% of the blood volume [2].

Unlike many other cells, mature red blood cells have no nuclei in humans and thus have a very flexible structure. Because of these flexible structures, they can easily reach everywhere through the blood vessels. The biconcave shape also provides a greater surface area across which gas exchange can occur, relative to its volume [3]. This flexible shape also limits the life of the cell. The red blood cell survives only an average of 120 days [4, 5]. In time, the membrane of the red blood cells becomes easily vulnerable and they are removed from the circulation by reticuloendothelial system macrophages mostly in the spleen. After phagocytosis, the hemoglobin is exposed. Macrophages remove the iron from hemoglobin for reutilization. Iron is bound to transferrin in the blood. The remaining parts of the hemoglobin are converted to bilirubin and given to the blood and then excreted into the bile by the liver.

2. Conclusion

Erythrocytes are the basis of life and erythrocyte evolution continues. We learned a lot, but there is still too much information to learn about erythrocytes. This book aims to reveal the latest developments related to "erythrocytes."

Author details

Anil Tombak
Department of Internal Medicine—Hematology, Mersin University Medical Faculty, Mersin, Turkey

*Address all correspondence to: aniltombak@mersin.edu.tr

References

[1] Mothlag SP, Zarejabad AM, Nasrabadi RG, Ahmadifar E, Molaee M. Haematology, morphology and blood cells characteristics of male and female Siamese fighting fish (*Betta splendens*). Comparative Clinical Pathology. 2012;**21**:15-21. DOI: 10.1007/s00580-010-1058-6

[2] Tombak A. Red blood cells and relation to thrombosis. In: Koopman-van Gemert AWMM, editor. Transfusion Medicine and Scientific Developments. IntechOpen; 2017. DOI: 10.5772/intechopen.69551

[3] Whelihan MF, Mann KG. The role of the red cell membrane in thrombin generation. Thrombosis Research. 2013;**131**:377-382. DOI: 10.1016/j.thromres.2013.01.023

[4] Franco RS. The measurement and importance of red cell survival. American Journal of Hematology. 2009;**84**(2):109-114. DOI: 10.1002/ajh.21298

[5] Korolnek T, Hamza I. Macrophages and iron trafficking at the birth and death of red cells. Blood. 2015;**125**(19):2893-2897. DOI: 10.1182/blood-2014-12-567776

Chapter 2

Erythrocyte Morphology and Its Disorders

Ademola Samson Adewoyin, Oluwafemi Adeyemi, Nosimot Omolola Davies and Ann Abiola Ogbenna

Abstract

Blood cell morphology is a key tool in laboratory haematology. Erythrocyte morphology points to possible aetiopathogenetic events in several primary and secondary haemopathies. Despite advances in medical technology and laboratory automation, red cell morphology remains a basic aspect of haematological evaluation. The human erythrocytes are discoid (bi-concave), about 7–8 μm (size of the nucleus of a small lymphocyte) in diameter, with a central area of pallor (which occupies a third of the red cell diameter) and is well haemoglobinised in the outer two thirds of the red cell diameters, without any inclusions. Deviations from the normal in terms of size, shape, colour, distribution or presence of inclusion bodies suggests possible disease processes. This chapter is therefore dedicated to morphologic description of the human erythrocytes, a study of possible abnormalities, its underlying pathophysiology and the associated differential diagnosis in humans.

Keywords: red cell, erythrocytes, morphology, haematology, red cell disorders, peripheral blood film

1. Introduction

Erythrocytes are the major cellular component of the circulating blood. Roughly, erythrocytes in circulation average about 5 million cells per cubic millimetres of blood. With an average life span of about 100–120 days, erythrocyte production and senescence is maintained in constant equilibrium. Any imbalances affecting production or destruction of red cells result in red cell disorder. In essence, red cells are maintained at a constant volume in the body, depending on several factors. Physiologic factors such as age, sex, altitude, smoking status or pregnancy account for slight inter-individual and intra-individual variations. Typically, there are different measures of red cell counts and they include red cell mass, red cell volume, red cell count, haematocrit and haemoglobin concentration. Red cell volume or mass is expected to fall within an interval of mean ± 2 SD within a specified population for a person's age, sex and race.

Beyond count anomalies (quantitative abnormalities), morphologic aberrations (qualitative abnormalities) are highly relevant in clinical evaluation of red cell diseases. Normally, a red cell has a round form, shaped like a disc, well-haemoglobinised cytoplasmic rim with a central pallor covering inner third of the red cell. Deviations in morphology (size, shape, colour, contents/inclusion or distribution) may be associated or perhaps diagnostic of disease entities. For instance, a blood picture with paucity of red cells, numerous red cell fragments, increased polychromatic red cells suggests a micro-angiopathy or fragmentation syndrome.

This chapter aims to discuss principles of red cell morphology, as well as describe red cells in terms of morphology, identify morphologic abnormalities associated with different disease conditions.

2. Principles of erythrocyte morphology

Circulating red cells are formed from bone marrow stem cells. Stem cells are pluripotent; they self-replicate and differentiate to specialized cells in circulation through different lineages. Red cells are formed from the myeloid stem cell lineage (colony forming unit—granulocytes, erythroid, myeloid and megakaryocytes). The earliest recognizable red cell precursor in the bone marrow is the pronormoblast. The pronormoblast undergoes series of maturation to become the orthochromatic normoblast. Upon extrusion of its nucleus, the late normoblast becomes the shift reticulocytes, which is released into the circulation. Finally, DNA remnants and other chromatin materials in the reticulocytes is removed by the pitting action of the spleen, hence the mature red cells.

Erythrocytes cannot be seen with the naked eyes. Typically, morphology of red cells is performed on peripheral blood smears, once there is an indication. Erythrocyte morphology is either indicated by a clinical request or laboratory flags. Examples of clinical indications for peripheral blood film/erythrocyte morphology are listed in **Table 1**.

Erythrocyte morphology may also be indicated when significant deviations from the normal are seen in the laboratory during blood work (full blood count) irrespective of a clinical request. For instance, a significantly reduced haemoglobin level with low MCV and raised RDW may suggest iron deficiency anaemia. This is an indication for red cell morphology and other ancillary investigation for iron deficiency.

Blood for peripheral blood film is collected through venipuncture. Anticoagulant of choice is the potassium EDTA. Specimens should be analysed as

A clinical request for a PBF may be prompted by the following indications:
• Unexplained anaemia, leucopenia or thrombocytopenia
• Unexplained leukocytosis, lymphocytosis or monocytosis
• Unexplained jaundice or haemolysis
• Features of congenital haemolytic anaemias such as splenomegaly, jaundice or bone pains
• Suspected chronic or acute myeloproliferative disease, e.g. Chronic myeloid leukaemia
• Suspected organ failure such as renal disease, liver failure
• Features of hyperviscosity syndrome as in paraproteinaemias, leukaemic hyperleucocytosis, polycythaemia
• Severe bacterial sepsis and parasitic infections
• Advanced malignancies with possible bone marrow involvement
• Suspected cases of nutritional anaemia
• Suspected chronic lymphoproliferative such as chronic lymphocytic leukaemia
• Advanced lymphoma with leukaemic spills
• Evaluation of disseminated intravascular coagulopathy and other red cell fragmentation syndromes

Table 1.
Clinical indications for peripheral blood film.

Cell component	Colour
Chromatin (including H-J bodies)	Purple
Cytoplasm with RNA and nuclear Remnants (e.g. polychromasia, basophilic stippling's)	In polychromatic red cells, RNA produces a blue colour, which offsets the pink colour imparting a purple tinge Basophilic stippling: appears as blue granules dispersed within the cytoplasm in a punctate appearance
Mature red cells	Pink

Table 2.
Romanowsky staining characteristics of red cell components.

soon as possible, preferably within 2 hours of blood collection. Samples not analysed immediately should be stored at 2–6°C in a refrigerator, or the blood smear should be made, dried and fixed, for subsequent staining with Romanowsky dyes.

Asides automated slide makers, the commonest method for preparation of peripheral blood film is the slide 'wedge' or push technique. This technique typically requires microscope slides, pipette/blood dropper, spreader slide and the blood specimen to be analysed. Standard precautions must be observed to prevent transmission of infectious pathogens such as human immunodeficiency virus and hepatitis viruses.

Quality control measures will include ensuring proper anticoagulant: blood ratio, sample processing/analysis within sample viability period and adequate mixing of the blood before smearing. Each slide must be labelled with at least two patient identifiers such as name and laboratory, and date of procedure. Once the smear is air-dried in about 5–10 minutes, fixation of the blood tissue is another very important step. Fixation helps to preserve the architecture of the cells, which ensures good morphology. A dried slide should be fixed within 4 hours of preparation, preferably in the first hour.

For routine morphology, the glass slides are stained with Romanowsky dyes. Romanowsky dyes are differential stains composed of both acidic and basic components. The acidic component is eosin and the basic part is azure B or polychrome methylene blue. Examples of Romanowsky stains include Leishman stain, Jenner, Wright stain, May-Grunwald-Giemsa stain and Giemsa stain. Generally, the eosin part of the dye binds to the basic component of the cell such as the haemoglobin molecules in the red cell and stains it pink. The basophilic part of the dye binds to the acidic component of the cells such as the nucleus and stains it blue. Other components of the cells appear in different colour shades that contrasts and compares with the dye. The term, azurophilic is used to describe a neutral to sky-blue colour shade. For instance, the cytoplasm of a neutrophil is described as azurophilic in colour. Furthermore, the characteristic staining quality of different red cell components is presented in **Table 2**.

Staining procedure and the stain contact time depends on the type of dye in use. Staining protocols are contained in standard laboratory texts and reagent manuals. Red cell morphology should be examined at the monolayer region of the film which is 2–4 × 10 fields from the feathered edge. In this place red cells are randomly distributed with most lying singly and only a few overlapping. If area is too thin, the RBCs will appear flat with no central pallor. If too thick, false rouleaux may be reported and morphology may be difficult to evaluate because red cells are packed.

3. Red cell morphologic disorders

The haemato-morphologist reviews the red cell morphology under the compound microscope and notes any significant abnormalities for reporting/diagnosis in light of patient clinical context. Red cell morphology is evaluated in terms of size, shape, colour, distribution and intra cytoplasmic inclusions. In general, red cells have a fairly uniform variation in size, with a red cell distribution width of 11–15% in normal individuals. Abnormal variations in sizes and shape are termed anisocytosis and poikilocytosis, respectively [1].

3.1 Anisocytosis

Normal red cells (normocytes) are about 7–8 μm in diameter [2]. Reduced size is termed microcytosis. Increase in red cell diameter above normal is called macrocytosis. Red cell sizes form the basis for morphologic or cytometric classification of anaemia. In terms of red cell size, anaemia could be described as microcytic, normocytic or macrocytic. Typically, the normal red cell size is adjudged by comparison with the nucleus of a small lymphocyte. The reference interval for mean red cell volume (MCV) is 80–95 fl [3, 4]. MCV >95 fl is termed macrocytic. While, red cell size <6 μm and/or MCV <80 fl is termed microcytic [5]. Differentials of microcytic anaemias include iron deficiency, thalassemias, sideroblastic anaemia and anaemia of chronic inflammation (20% of cases). Further test such as serum ferritin, total iron binding capacity (TIBC), haemoglobin electrophoresis with quantification helps to differentiate microcytic anaemia [4, 6]. For instance, low serum ferritin, raised TIBC and raised RDW is expected in iron deficiency. A normal or elevated red cell counts with little red cell size variation (RDW) in the presence of microcytosis is suggestive of a thalassaemia.

Normocytic anaemia occurs in acute blood loss, marrow aplasia, anaemia of chronic disease (80% of cases) and anaemias of endocrine origin. Macrocytosis may be oval or round, with specific casual relationships. Oval macrocytes are seen in megaloblastic anaemias (folate/cobalamin deficiencies), myelodysplastic syndrome and drug therapies such as hydroxyurea [7]. Round macrocytes are seen in liver disease and excess alcohol use. MCV may appear falsely normal with the haematology analyser in combined substrate deficiency states. However, the blood picture will reveal marked anisopoikilocytosis. The red cell distribution width (RDW) is a calculated parameter and it measures the individual size variability (heterogeneity) of the red cells. RDW is the percentage coefficient of variation of the individual red cell volumes enumerated by the particle counter [8]. RDW normally ranges between 11.5 and 15.5%. For interpretation purposes, raised RDW is seen in iron deficiency anaemia, megaloblastic anaemia (folate and cobalamin deficiency), haemolytic anaemia, recent blood transfusion, hereditary spherocytosis and sickle cell syndromes [8, 9]. RDW is useful in interpreting apparently normal MCV since it will be quite high in combined micronutrient deficiency state.

3.2 Poikilocytosis

Shape abnormalities, otherwise called poikilocytes are useful pointers to specific diagnosis. It is important to note that poikilocytosis may also occur in vitro (artefactual causes). It is therefore necessary to ensure adequate precautions in reducing pre-analytic and intra-analytic errors that affects morphology. As a reminder, the following quality control measures apply in blood film morphology:

- Blood specimens for PBF are best collected in EDTA bottles through venipuncture.

- Optimal blood: anticoagulant ratio should be observed.

- Samples should be dispatched immediately to the haematology laboratory. Prolonged delay in analysis allows for cellular degeneration, pseudo-thrombocytopenia and artefactual changes [10].

- Blood specimens for morphology are best analysed within 2 hours of collection.

Poikilocytes are categorized as either spiculated or non-spiculated. Spiculated red cells have at least one pointed projection from the cell surface. Examples of spiculated poikilocytes are burr cells, schistocytes (red cell fragments), irreversibly sickled red cells (drepanocytes), acanthocytes and tear drop red cells (dacrocytes). Non-spiculated poikilocytes include target cells, ovalocytes and stomatocytes. Various mechanical, biochemical and molecular mechanisms underlie pathologic changes in red cell shape. Some occur as a result of disturbances in the haematopoietic system. Target cells have an area of central haemoglobinization (termed hyperchromic bull eyes) surrounded by a halo of pallor. Increased red cell surface area to volume ratio in target cells is due to its redundant membrane, which gives rise to the targetoid shape. Target cells (**Figure 1**) are seen in sickle haemoglobinopathies, thalassemias, iron deficiency and post splenectomy state. Tear drop red cells (**Figure 2**) results from abnormal spleen or bone marrow pathology such as primary myelofibrosis when the red cells stretch out in order to navigate its way into the periphery or as a result of stretching from the pitting action of the spleen, when red cells with inclusions such as Heinz bodies navigates the splenic cords into the sinuses [5].

Stomatocytes have a fish mouth appearance (slit-like central pallor). They are mostly due to increased red cell permeability, resulting in increased volume. Stomatocytes may be inherited or acquired. Hereditary stomatocytosis is seen in Rh null phenotype. Acquired stomatocytosis is mostly seen with recent excessive alcohol and typically resolves within 2 weeks of alcohol withdrawal. When artefactual, stomatocytes are usually <10% of the red cell population. As the name implies, irreversibly sickled red cells (**Figure 1**) are seen in sickle syndromes. The primary event is intra-erythrocytic haemoglobin precipitation (gelation), with resultant formation of tactoids, which deforms the discoid red cell to sickle or crescent morphology [11]. Burr cells are seen in renal failure and may be artefactual. Artefactual red

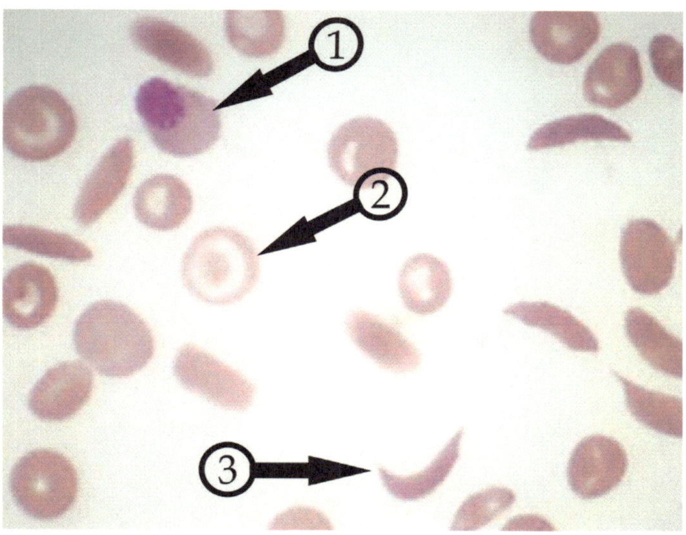

Figure 1.
(1) Nucleated red cell, (2) target cell, and (3) irreversibly sickled red cell.

cells may be caused by poor fixation and high humidity in the laboratory ambience. Artefactual tear drop cells should be suspected if the tails line up in the same direction. **Table 3** itemizes common poikilocytes and its differentials [1, 5, 12–15].

3.3 Anisochromia/polychromasia

Anisochromia depicts increased or decreased haemoglobinization of the red cells. In hypochromic red cells, the central pallor exceeds one third of the diameter. Hypochromia usually follows microcytosis, as seen in iron deficiency states. Hyperchromia (increased haemoglobinisation) is associated with shape abnormalities such as (micro)-spherocytes and sickled red cells. Increased haemoglobinization obliterates central pallor. Occasionally, severe hypochromia is associated with macrocytic red cells, termed leptocytes. Leptocytes are seen in severe iron deficiency, thalassemia and liver diseases [14]. Polychromasia on PBF suggests in-vivo reticulocytosis. Literally, polychromasia means 'many colours', i.e. the red cells bear another shade of colour than pink (eosinophilic). Polychromatic red cells are macrocytic (young red cells) and have a bluish tinge. The blue tinge denotes the presence of rRNA which eventually undergo the pitting action of the spleen to become mature circulating red cells [1]. Normally, polychromatic red cells are not obvious on PBF—adult reticulocyte population is about 0.5–2.5% [3]. However, polychromatic red cells in excess of 1–2% in the periphery should be considered significant since normal daily rate of red cell turnover is about 1–2% [16]. In situations of acute haemorrhage, haemolysis, and high altitude, hypoxia induces increased erythroid activity, hence polychromasia. Polychromasia is also seen in extramedullary haemopoiesis due to myeloid metaplasia in reticulo-endothelial tissue. Following haematinic therapy, polychromatic red cells are seen as a response to treatment of micronutrient deficiency [1].

Similarly, in severe situations causing marrow stress, nucleated red cells (erythroblastosis) exit the bone marrow prematurely in order to compensate. Notable causes of erythroblastosis (or normoblastemia) include severe anaemia, asplenic/hyposplenic state as in sickle cell disease, severe hypoxia, marrow replacements or infiltrations and extramedullary haemopoiesis [17, 18]. In neonates, nucleated red cells are normally seen in the periphery [15].

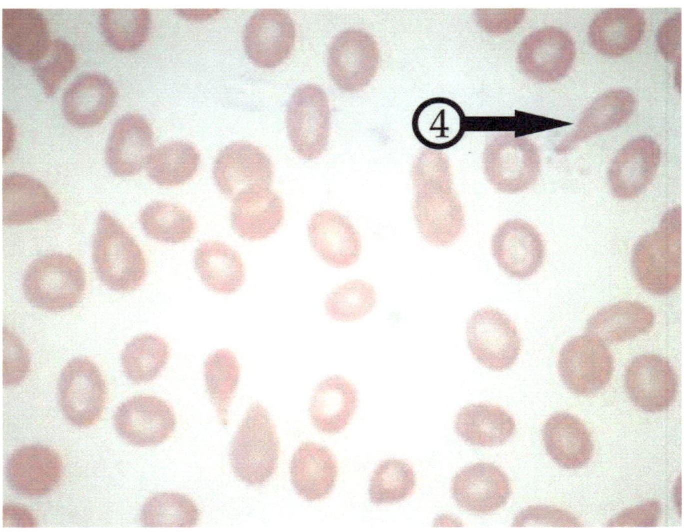

Figure 2.
(4) Tear drop red cell.

Red cell shapes	Differential diagnosis
Irreversibly sickled red cells (drepanocytes)	Sickle cell syndromes (SS, SC, S-β-thalassemia)
Target red cells (codocytes) Target cells (codocytes, Mexican hat cells)	Sickle cell disease, haemoglobin C trait, haemoglobin CC disease, thalassemia's, iron deficiency, liver disease (cholestasis), asplenia
Fragmented red cells (schistocytes, helmet cells, keratocytes)	Thrombotic micro-angiopathic haemolytic anaemias such as disseminated intravascular coagulopathy (DIC), thrombotic thrombocytopenic purpura, haemolytic uraemic syndrome.
Pencil cells	Iron deficiency
Stomatocytes	Artefact (due to slow drying in humid environment), liver disease, alcoholism, Rh-null disease, obstructive lung disease
Elliptocytes	Hereditary elliptocytosis (>25%)
Bite cells (degmacytes)	G6PD deficiency, oxidative stress, unstable haemoglobin's, congenital Heinz body anaemia
Basket cells (half ghost cells/ blister cells)	Oxidant damage, G6PD deficiency, unstable haemoglobin's
Spherocytes	Hereditary spherocytosis, ABO incompatibility, autoimmune haemolytic anaemia (warm antibody type), severe burns
Teardrop red cell (dacrocytes, lacrymocytes)	Idiopathic myelofibrosis, myelophthisic anaemia, thalassemia's

Table 3.
Red cell shape anomalies and associated diseases.

3.4 Other red cell abnormalities

Other morphologic abnormalities include presence of inclusion bodies and pathologic distribution of red cells on the smear. A mature erythrocyte lacks inclusion bodies. Red cell inclusion bodies include nuclear products RNA/DNA, haemoglobin or iron pigments. Some, such as haemoglobin H inclusions and Heinz bodies can only be appreciated with supravital staining. Red cell inclusions result from oxidant stress, severe infections and dyserythropoiesis (maturation defects). Basophilic stipplings or punctuate basophilia are denatured RNA fragments dispersed within the cytoplasm. Basophilic stipplings may be fine, blue stipplings or coarse granules. They are non-specific and are generally related to disorders in haem biosynthetic pathways [1, 19]. Differentials include haemoglobinopathies (thalassemias), lead or arsenic poisoning, unstable haemoglobins, severe infections, sideroblastic anaemia, megaloblastic anaemia and a rare inherited condition, pyrimidine 5′ nucleotidase deficiency [1, 10, 20].

Clinically insignificant, fine basophilic stippling may be associated with polychromasia/accelerated erythropoiesis/reticulocytosis. Coarse stipplings are clinically significant and indicates impaired haemoglobin synthesis as seen in megaloblastic anaemia, thalassemias, sideroblastic anaemias and lead poisoning [1, 19]. Unlike other basophilic inclusions such as Howell jolly bodies and Pappenheimer bodies which tend to be displaced to the periphery, basophilic stipplings are diffusely dispersed throughout the red cell cytoplasm. Howell jolly bodies (**Figure 3**) are DNA remnants seen in post-splenectomy patients, anatomical or functional asplenia. Siderotic granules or Pappenheimer bodies appear purple on Romanowsky stain, blue on Perl's stain and are seen in disorders of iron utilization like sideroblastic anaemias.

Parasites such as *Plasmodium* spp. or *Babesia* spp. may also be seen on peripheral blood smear [21]. Both parasites invade the red cells. Their identification requires

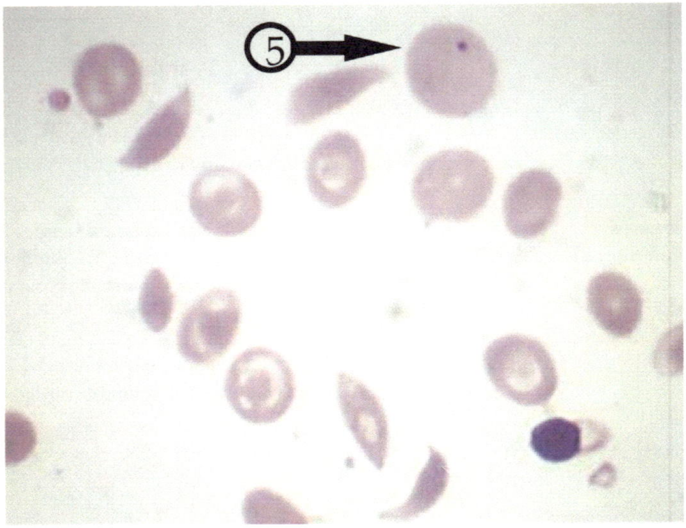

Figure 3.
(5) Howell Jolly body (in a 36-year-old lady with sickle cell disease).

some level of knowledge and experience. Several species of *Plasmodium* spp. exist. *Plasmodium* spp. may exist in different forms such as ring forms (trophozoites), gametocytes and schizonts. *Babesia* spp. appear in small ring forms (like *Plasmodium falciparum*) but schizonts and gametocytes are not formed [1, 21]. Unlike *Plasmodium* spp., *Babesia* spp. do not produce pigments. However, *Babesia* spp. may appear in groups outside the erythrocyte. Clinical history and travel history is also helpful in differentiating the two parasites. Other red cell inclusions such as Heinz bodies and haemoglobin H inclusions can only be appreciated with supravital staining (reticulocyte preparations). Heinz bodies are denatured haemoglobin (seen in oxidant injury, G6PD deficiency). Haemoglobin H inclusions are seen in alpha-thalassemias giving rise to the characteristic 'golf ball' appearance of the erythrocytes [1, 11, 12].

Rouleaux formation refers to stacking of red cells like coins in a single file. Rouleaux is seen in hyperproteinaemias. Elevated plasma fibrinogen or globulins reduces the zeta potential (repulsive force) between circulating red cells, facilitating their stacking effect. Rouleaux is associated with myeloma/paraproteinaemias, other plasma cell disorders as well as B cell lymphomas. On the other hand, agglutination refers to clumping or aggregation of red cells into clusters or masses and is usually antibody mediated [1]. Agglutination of red cells may be seen in cold haemagglutinin disease and Waldenstrom's macroglobulinaemia [1, 11]. Agglutination is associated with falsely reduced red cell count and high MCV. Pre warming the specimen with heating block helps to disperse the red cells prior to making of a blood smear and automated cell counts.

4. Conclusion

Red cell morphology is crucial in evaluating anaemias and several blood disorders. Good quality smear, with proper Romanowsky/special staining, coupled with the expertise of an haemato-morphologists (haematologists/haematology pathologists) remains highly valuable in patient care.

Author details

Ademola Samson Adewoyin[1*], Oluwafemi Adeyemi[2], Nosimot Omolola Davies[1] and Ann Abiola Ogbenna[1]

1 College of Medicine, University of Lagos, Lagos, Nigeria

2 University of Benin Teaching Hospital, Benin City, Nigeria

*Address all correspondence to: doctordemola@gmail.com

References

[1] Jones KW. Evaluation of cell morphology and introduction to platelet and white blood cell morphology. In: Harmening D, editor. Clinical Hematology and Fundamentals of Hemostasis. Philadelphia; 2009. pp. 93-116

[2] Wickramasinghe SN, Erber WN, editors. Normal blood cells. In: Blood and Bone Marrow Pathology. Elsevier; 2011

[3] Hoffbrand AV, PAH M, Pettit JE, editors. Erythropoiesis and general aspects of anaemia. In: Essential Haematology. 2011. pp. 15-32

[4] Perkins S. Diagnosis of anaemia. In: Kjeldsberg CR, editor. Practical Diagnosis of Hematologic Disorders. Singapore: ASCP Press; 2006. p. 16

[5] Glassy E. Color Atlas of Haematology. An Illustrated Field Guide Based on Proficiency Testing. Northfield, Illinois: College of American Pathologists; 1998

[6] Ogedegbe HO. Anemias: A clinical perspective. Laboratory Medicine. 2004;**3**:177-185

[7] Hoffbrand AV. Megaloblastic anaemia. In: Victor Hoffbrand A, Catovsky D, Edward GD, et al., editors. Postgraduate Haematology. West Sussex: Wiley-Blackwell; 2011

[8] Buttarello M, Plebani M. Automated blood cell counts: State of the art. American Journal of Clinical Pathology. 2008;**130**:104-116

[9] Briggs C. Quality counts: New parameters in blood cell counting. International Journal of Laboratory Hematology. 2009;**31**:277-297

[10] Bain BJ. Diagnosis from the blood smear. The New England Journal of Medicine. 2005;**353**:498-507

[11] Madigan C, Malik P. Pathophysiology and therapy for haemoglobinopathies. Part 1: Sickle cell disease. Expert Reviews in Molecular Biology. 2006;**8**:1-23

[12] Ford J. Red blood cell morphology. International Journal of Laboratory Haematology. 2013;**35**:351-357

[13] Adewoyin AS, Nwogoh B. Peripheral blood film: A review. Annals of Ibadan Postgraduate Medicine;**12**:71-79

[14] Bain BJ. Blood cell morphology in health and disease. In: Dacie and Lewis Practical Heaematology. 11th ed. 2012. pp. 69-100

[15] Longo DL. Atlas of haematology and analysis of peripheral blood smear. In: Haematology and Oncology. pp. 57-68

[16] Koury MJ. Red cell production and kinetics. In: Simon TL et al., editors. Rossi's Principles of Transfusion Medicine. West Sussex: Wiley-Blackwell; 2009. pp. 17-28

[17] Constantino BT, Cogionis B. Nucleated RBCs–significance in the peripheral blood film. Laboratory Medicine. 2000;**31**:223-229

[18] Akhtar S, Mahure S. Nuance of nucleated rbcs (normoblastemia) in peripheral blood film. Panacea Journal of Medical Science. 2015;**5**:7-13

[19] Hays T, Jamieson B. Atlas of Pediatric Peripheral Blood Smears. 1st ed. Abbott Laboratories; 2008

[20] Marinaki AM, Escuredo E, Duley JA, Simmonds HA, Amici A, et al. Genetic basis of hemolytic anemia caused by pyrimidine 5' nucleotidase deficiency. Blood. 2001;**97**:3327-3332

[21] Moody AH, Chiodini PL. Methods for the detection of blood parasites. Clinical and Laboratory Haematology. 2000;**22**:189-202

Chapter 3

Red Blood Cells Actively Contribute to Blood Coagulation and Thrombus Formation

Ingolf Bernhardt, Mauro C. Wesseling, Duc Bach Nguyen and Lars Kaestner

Abstract

The chapter describes the likely molecular mechanisms leading to the aggregation of human red blood cells (RBCs) under conditions of physiological coagulation when prostaglandin E_2 (PGE_2) or lysophosphatidic acid (LPA) is released from activated platelets and under pathophysiological conditions, in particular thrombi formation in sickle cell disease when patients are in a vaso-occlusive crisis. In both scenarios cation channels are activated. This leads to an increase of the free intracellular Ca^{2+} concentration resulting in an activation of the lipid scramblase, which in turn mediates a movement of phosphatidylserine (PS) from the inner to the outer membrane leaflet. In addition, the increased Ca^{2+} concentration leads to the activation of the Gardos channel. Experiments suggesting this mechanism have been performed with fluorescence microscopy, flow cytometry as well as single-cell force spectroscopy. The Ca^{2+}-triggered RBC aggregation force has been identified to be close to 100 pN, a value large enough to play a significant role during thrombus formation or in pathological situations.

Keywords: red blood cells, intracellular Ca^{2+} concentration, phosphatidylserine, cation channels, lipid scramblase, thrombus formation

1. Introduction

It is well known that phospholipids are asymmetrically distributed in the cell membrane of most, if not all, living cells. Sphingomyelin (SM) and phosphatidylcholine (PC) are located predominantly in the outer leaflet of the membrane bilayer, while phosphatidylserine (PS) and phosphatidylethanolamine (PE) are located mostly in the inner leaflet [1] as depicted in **Figure 1A**. **Figure 1B** shows the possible movements of phospholipids from one leaflet of the membrane to the other one (for explanation see text below).

The distribution of the membrane phospholipids is realised by three main proteins: flippase [4], floppase and scramblase [2, 5, 6]. The flippase (also named aminophospholipid translocase (APLT)) transports relatively quickly (in some minutes) PS, and a bit slower PE, from the outer to the inner membrane leaflet. The floppase transports PC and SM in the opposite direction, i.e. from the inner to the outer membrane leaflet [2]. The flippase and floppase are ATP-dependent

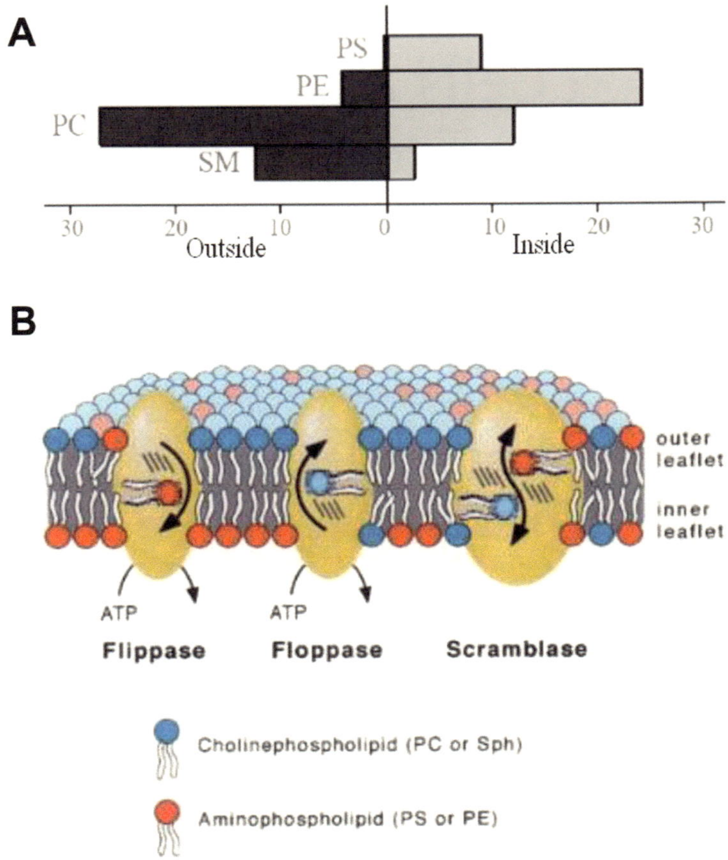

Figure 1.
(A) The asymmetric distribution of phospholipids in the human red cell membrane. Abbreviations: SM, sphingomyelin; PC, phosphatidylcholine; PE, phosphatidylethanolamine; PS, phosphatidylserine. (B) Transporter-controlled exchange of phospholipids between both lipid leaflets of the cell membrane. Unidirectional phospholipid transport by flippase is directed inwards, whereas floppase promotes outward directed transport. Both transporters are ATP-dependent and frequently move phospholipids against their respective concentration gradients. For example, aminophospholipid translocase (flippase) rapidly shuttles PS and PE from outer to inner leaflet, while ABCC1 (floppase) moves both choline phospholipids and aminophospholipids more slowly towards the outer leaflet. The concerted action of both transporters is thought to create a dynamic asymmetric steady state, in which the outer monolayer is rich in choline phospholipids, whereas aminophospholipids predominantly occupy the inner leaflet. Bidirectional phospholipid transport is catalysed by a scramblase, the activation of which may occur following Ca^{2+} increase. Since scramblase activity moves all major phospholipid classes back and forth between the two leaflets, it promotes the collapse of membrane phospholipid asymmetry with appearance of PS at the cells' outer surface. Panel (A) is modified from [2], and (B) is reproduced from [3].

and transport the phospholipids against their respective concentration gradients. The structure of the flippase has been published recently [7]. The scramblase is ATP-independent and activated by an increasing intracellular Ca^{2+} concentration in human red blood cells (RBCs) [8]. The scramblase has been identified recently as a member of the TMEM16 protein family, and the crystal structure was published [9]. The activity of the three proteins is shown in **Figure 1B**. PS exposure on the outer leaflet of the cell membrane has been described as a marker for apoptosis in nucleated cells [5]. Although the programmed cell death of RBCs is still under discussion, these cells show some signs of apoptosis such as PS exposure, membrane blebbing and vesicle formation [10]. This process was denominated eryptosis by Lang et al. [11]. However, the use of this term is very controversial and finally not recommended [12].

Based on findings showing a correlation between decreased haematocrit and longer bleeding times [13] and experiments of Andrews and Low [14], an active role of RBCs in thrombus formation has been proposed [14]. Kaestner et al. suggested a more detailed signalling cascade based on Ca^{2+} uptake via a non-selective cation channel that could be activated by prostaglandin E_2 (PGE_2) and/or lysophosphatidic acid (LPA) [15–17]. Recent considerations suggest more complicated signalling cascades to be involved [18, 19], including the participation of the mechanosensitive channel Piezo1 [20, 21].

Although it is known that LPA induces PS exposure on the outer membrane leaflet in RBCs, there are conflicting reports about the mechanism. While Chung et al. [22] claim that it is a totally Ca^{2+}-independent process, we showed that Ca^{2+} alone is sufficient to induce PS exposure in human RBCs [23]. Woon et al. found that an increase of the intracellular Ca^{2+} level in RBCs results in the exposure of PS to the outer membrane leaflet due to the activation of the scramblase and inhibition of the flippase [24]. Protein kinase Cα (PKCα) has been also described to be involved in the PS exposure on RBCs [22, 25, 26]. A further discussion follows below.

An interesting model for lipid studies we consider below is sheep RBCs since it is known that these cells have a completely different phospholipid distribution in the membrane. Like in human RBCs, PS and PE are distributed in the inner membrane leaflet. In contrast, the sheep RBC (like all bovine RBC) membrane does not contain any PC, and the outer layer consists exclusively of SM [27, 28].

2. Stimulation of intracellular Ca^{2+} increase in human RBCs

PGE_2 and LPA are local mediators released by platelets after their activation within the coagulation cascade. PGE_2 can be even released by the RBCs themselves under conditions of mechanical stress [29]. We were able to show that the addition of both mediators to suspensions of human RBCs leads to an increase of the intracellular free Ca^{2+} concentration in these cells. In the case of PGE_2 (0.1 nM), 45% of the RBCs responded with increased Ca^{2+} content; in the case of LPA (5 μM), nearly all cells reacted [17, 30] but still showed a strong heterogeneity in the time course and the intensity of the response [31].

The identity of the Ca^{2+} entry was proposed to be channel-mediated; on the one hand, the $Ca_V2.1$-channel [32] and on the other hand the non-selective voltage dependent cation channel [17] were suggested. While the activation of $Ca_V2.1$ was linked to protein kinase C (PKC) activity [33], we could show that $Ca_V2.1$ and PKC belong to different signalling branches [18].

However, in a series of papers utilising fluorescence microscopy and flow cytometry, we could link PKCα activity and Ca^{2+} entry [30, 34].

The above described effect is probably mediated by a specific pathway rather than a non-specific leak since the Ca^{2+} entry shows a clear dose-response relationship towards the LPA concentration [35]. For a recent review about Ca^{2+} channels in human RBCs, see [36].

Another known port for Ca^{2+} entry that is likely to have some pathophysiological relevance is the NMDA-receptor. Among the RBCs, NMDA-receptors were first identified in rat RBCs [37] but later also in human precursor cells as well as in circulating RBCs [38]. NMDA-receptors are cation channels permeable to Ca^{2+} and can be activated by homocysteine and homocysteic acid [39].

To extend on this, **Figure 2** provides an overview of the current knowledge about Ca^{2+} entry and the major cellular consequences in different pathophysiological conditions.

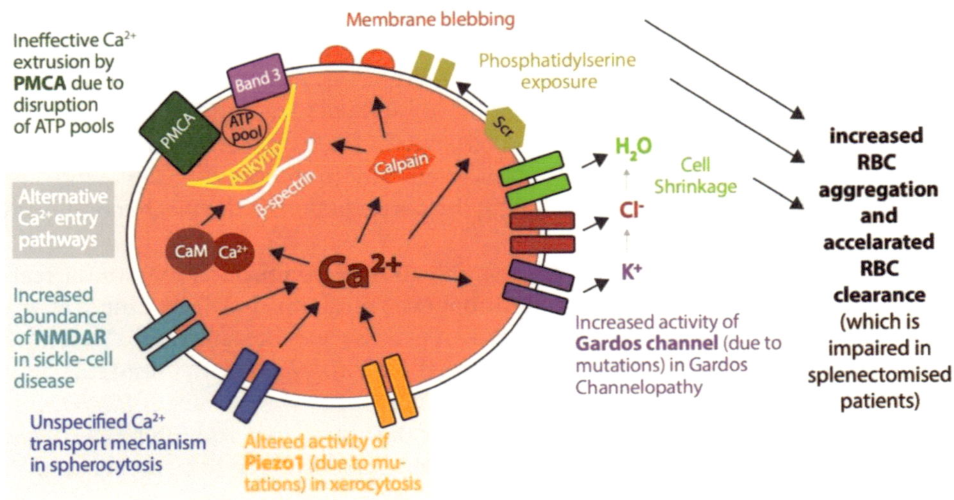

Figure 2.
Proposed mechanisms leading to increased intracellular Ca^{2+} levels in diseased RBCs. Alternative or cumulating Ca^{2+} entry pathways are highlighted with grey background: increased abundance of NMDA-receptors (NMDAR), e.g. in sickle cell disease; altered activity of Piezo1, e.g. in hereditary xerocytosis; increased activity of the Gardos channel, e.g. in Gardos Channelopathy; or unspecified Ca^{2+} transport mechanisms. Additionally, ineffective extrusion of Ca^{2+} due to disruption of ATP pools fuelling the plasma membrane Ca^{2+} ATPase (PMCA) can contribute. Several downstream processes follow Ca^{2+} overload in RBCs, e.g. activation of calmodulin by formation of the Ca^{2+}-calmodulin complex (Ca-CaM) and activation of calpain, thereby loosening the cytoskeletal structure; activation of the scramblase (Scr) leading to exposure of phosphatidylserine on the outer leaflet of the membrane; activation of the Gardos channel followed by the efflux of K^+, Cl^- and H_2O; and consecutive cell shrinkage. All these processes may lead to an increased RBC aggregation and/or accelerated RBC clearance, which is impaired when patients are splenectomised. This figure is modified from Hertz et al. [40].

3. Increased intracellular Ca^{2+} content of human RBCs results in an activation of the scramblase

The PS exposure on the outer membrane leaflet of RBCs was studied for LPA-treated cells using fluorescence microscopy. It has been shown that the number of annexin V-positive cells (i.e. cells showing PS exposure) after LPA treatment in the presence of Ca^{2+} is about 35% [30].

Experiments have also been carried out after treating the RBCs with LPA or the PKC-activator PMA but in the absence of extracellular Ca^{2+} (presence of 1 mM EGTA). In the case of LPA, we did not find significant differences between treatment and control conditions (without activation) regarding PS exposure on human RBCs. Only in the case of PMA treatment, about 50% of RBCs showed PS exposure in the absence of Ca^{2+} (compared to about 80% in the presence of Ca^{2+}). The data obtained for control conditions in the presence of Ca^{2+} were not significantly different from the data of the control conditions in the absence of Ca^{2+} [30].

It is evident that for stimulation with the phorbol ester PMA, there is no correlation between the number of cells showing an elevated Ca^{2+} content and the induced PS exposure, because it is known that PMA activates PKCα also in the absence of Ca^{2+}.

Furthermore we like to state that the threshold for the forward scatter in the flow cytometry measurements was set in a way to make sure that only the events based on the size of intact cells were counted. This was of importance since we realised the formation of micro-vesicles after treatment with LPA as well as with PMA, which is in agreement with findings reported before [41, 42]. Calpain, a Ca^{2+}-dependent proteolytic enzyme, cleaves spectrin and actin, leading to cytoskeleton breakdown [43–45] and therefore could be involved in the vesiculation process.

The findings that Ca^{2+} content and PS exposure do not correlate in all cells were further supported by confocal fluorescence microscopy, where double-labelling experiments (for intracellular Ca^{2+} and PS in the outer membrane leaflet) have been carried out. The results of the LPA treatment showed that most of the cells have an elevated Ca^{2+} content and depict a PS exposure. However, some cells are displaying an increased Ca^{2+} level, but no PS exposure, whereas other cells externalise PS without having a higher Ca^{2+} content.

In the case of PMA treatment, PS exposure without high Ca^{2+} content is more pronounced, which is not surprising since PMA is an artificial compound, which activates conventional PKCs without the otherwise necessary presence of Ca^{2+}.

The percentage of RBCs showing PS exposure after activation with LPA or PMA is significantly reduced after inhibition of the scramblase using the specific inhibitor R5421 [34]. It is also significantly reduced after the inhibition of the PKCα using chelerythrine chloride or calphostin C. The inhibitory effect is more pronounced when the scramblase and the PKCα are inhibited simultaneously [34].

Based on our experiments, it seems reasonable to assume that at least three different mechanisms could be responsible for the PS exposure on RBCs:

- The first mechanism is related to the Ca^{2+}-stimulated scramblase activation (and flippase inhibition) [4, 8, 10, 11, 47]. This effect involves the activation of the ω-agatoxin-TK-sensitive, $Ca_V2.1$-like (P/Q-type) Ca^{2+} channel [33].

- The second mechanism involves the PKCα, which can be directly activated by PMA. It has been reported that PKCα is involved in the PS exposure in human RBCs [25, 26]. In addition, it has been shown that LPA activates in human RBCs both the PKCα (Ca^{2+}-dependent) and the PKCζ (Ca^{2+}-independent) [22]. Whether there is a direct activation of the scramblase in human RBCs by PKCα and/or PKCζ remains to be proofed. The more pronounced effect of PS exposure observed after treatment of RBCs with PMA as compared to LPA can be explained by assuming that PMA activates all available PKCα, whereas LPA stimulation triggers a signalling cascade [46] resulting only in partial activation of the PKCα pool.

- The third mechanism is the enhanced lipid flop caused by LPA [30]. This mechanism is the only one in sheep RBCs suggesting the absence of scramblase activity in these cells [30].

To consider a possible effect of cell volume alteration on PS exposure, experiments have been carried out where the physiological solution was replaced by a solution containing 150 mM KCl plus 2.5 mM NaCl instead of 145 mM NaCl plus 7.5 mM KCl. Under these conditions of a high extracellular KCl concentration, an opening of the Ca^{2+}-dependent K^+ channel (Gardos channel) does not result in a KCl loss and accompanying cell shrinkage. Based on this strategy, it has been found that a substantial part of the PS exposure in the presence of LPA is caused by the volume decrease.

It remains to be elucidated why, in the experiments reported above, some cells are displaying an increased Ca^{2+} level, but no PS exposure, whereas other cells externalise PS without having a higher Ca^{2+} content. In that context, we carried out single-labelling experiments (fluo-4 for intracellular Ca^{2+} and annexin V-FITC for exposed PS) and focussed on the shape of RBCs using also a fluorescence microscope. The obtained results are presented in **Figure 3**.

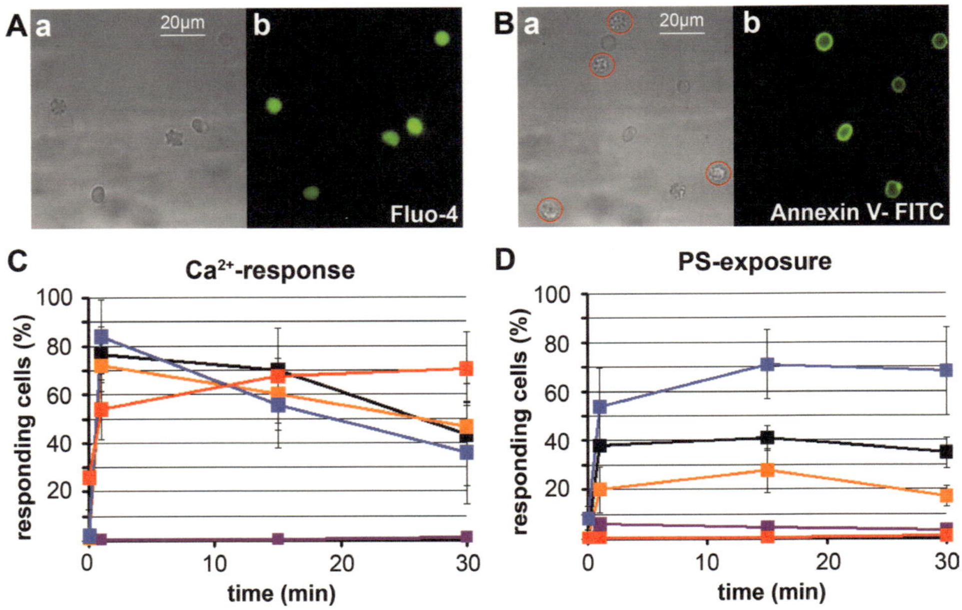

Figure 3.
Human RBC shapes after 2.5 µM LPA stimulation. Transmitted light (left) and fluorescence images (right) of RBCs. (A) Intracellular Ca^{2+} content detected using fluo-4, (B) PS exposure detecting using annexin V-FITC. (C, D) Flow cytometric analysis of responding cells after LPA stimulation in different solutions correlate with predominant cell shapes. Predominantly discocytes, physiological solution (black); predominantly echinocytes, low ionic strength solution + DIDS (red) and physiological solution + DIDS (orange); predominantly stomatocytes or discocytes, low ionic strength solution (blue); physiological solution at pH 5.6 (violet).

In **Figure 3Aa** one can see different cell shapes in the transmitted light image for LPA stimulation. However, the corresponding fluorescence image (**Figure 3Ab**) does not show differences of the increased Ca^{2+} content comparing RBCs with different shapes. The situation changes when analysing the PS exposure of the RBCs with different shapes (**Figure 3B**). Again, RBCs with different shapes can be seen (**Figure 3Ba**), but in the case of PS exposure, the cell shape seems to play a significant role. Some echinocytes can be seen in the transmitted light images (red circles in **Figure 3Ba**). Almost all of them lack PS exposure (corresponding fluorescence image in **Figure 3Bb**). Only one echinocyte showing PS exposure can be observed. The explanation of such an effect could be based on the bilayer couple hypothesis. If an echinocyte is formed, the outer membrane leaflet is already extended compared with the inner membrane leaflet. It means that any process of externalisation of a membrane lipid located mainly in the inner membrane leaflet is hindered. In addition we carried out experiments where we transferred the RBCs to different solutions as shown in **Figure 3C and D**. The RBC shapes, which predominantly occur in these solutions, are also indicated in **Figure 3**. Again, the PS exposure is lowest in solution where one can expect mostly echinocytes although the Ca^{2+} content is increased (red curves in **Figure 3**). The PS exposure of RBCs can be small also in solution where cells predominantly occur with the shape of discocytes or stomatocytes, however, in this case only in solutions where the increase of the intracellular Ca^{2+} content is prevented, e.g. physiological solution of low pH (5.6, see violet curves in **Figure 3**).

Furthermore, we carried out double-labelling experiments (X-Rhod-1 for intracellular Ca^{2+} and annexin V-FITC for exposed PS) and investigated the RBCs using a fluorescence microscope. The obtained results are presented in **Figure 4**. One RBC (indicated with white arrow in all panels of **Figure 4**) shows an increased intracellular Ca^{2+} content, but the cell suddenly disappeared from the transmitted light image

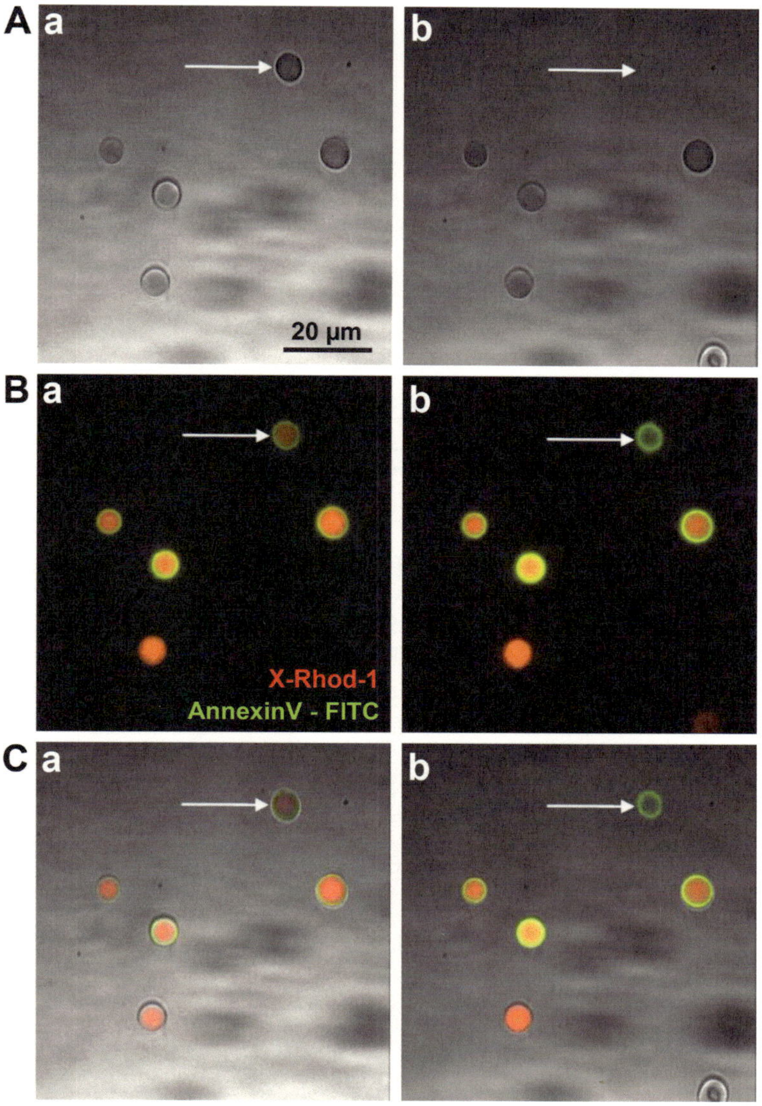

Figure 4.
RBCs were stimulated with lysophosphatidic acid, and panels (A) depict images 1 min after the start of the stimulation and panels (B) 1.5 min after the beginning of the stimulation. Panel (A) shows wide-field images and panel (B) confocal sections of the fluorescent biomarkers X-Rhod-1 (a Ca^{2+} indicator) and FITC-labelled annexin V (for PS detection). Panel (C) is an overlay of panels (A) and (B). The white arrow points to a cell that lysed after capturing images (a), i.e. in images (b) it's a ghost.

(**Figure 4Ab**). However, PS exposure of this cell still can be seen (**Figure 4Bb**). It can be assumed that this RBC lysed, i.e. we see the remaining membrane structure (a ghost) and the Ca^{2+}-sensitive fluorescent dye diffused out of the cell.

A different behaviour of RBCs depending on the age of the cell has been controversially discussed. Therefore, we performed additional short-time incubation experiments, comparable to the experiments carried out by Nguyen et al. [30], with RBCs separated in five fractions with different cell age according to the method of Lutz et al. [47]. The intracellular Ca^{2+} content and PS exposure at the outer membrane leaflet of human RBCs with different age have been investigated using, e.g. LPA stimulation. Here we present a reanalysis of these already published data [48]. Interestingly, the percentage of RBCs showing increased Ca^{2+} content and PS

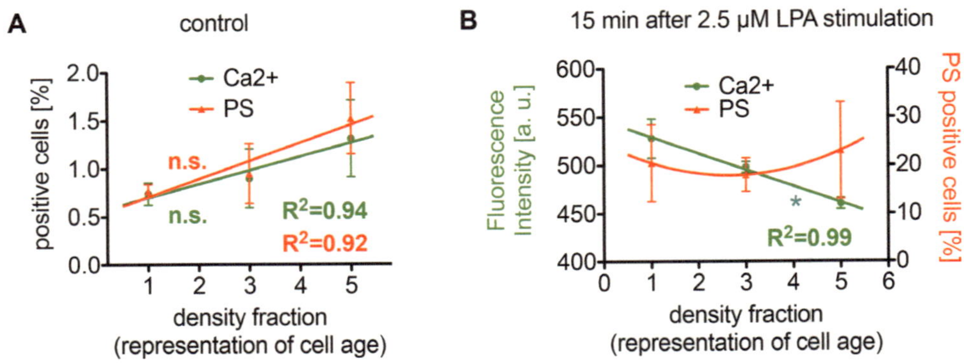

Figure 5.
*Reanalysis of data initially presented in [48]. In the original publication, only two fractions were compared with each other, while here we followed the approach to plot (and analyse) the measured effect in dependence of the cell age. (A) presents the situation under control conditions (without stimulation) and (B) the after 15 min stimulation with LPA ($p < 0.5$ is marked with *).*

exposure depict a linear behaviour in dependence of cell age with a very good regression, R^2 of 0.94 and 0.92, respectively, as outlined in **Figure 5A**. However, the slope of this linear regression failed to be significantly different from zero.

After stimulation of the RBCs with LPA, the situation is even more complex. **Figure 5B** depicts the situation after 15 min of LPA stimulation. While the Ca^{2+} concentration seems to relate inversely proportional to RBC age, PS-positive cells show a rather quadratic dependence on cell age. This is in contradiction to earlier investigations we performed on mouse RBCs [31]. Although we cannot completely resolve the situation part of the explanation might be caused in the detection technique: While microscopy is a rather gentle approach, in flow cytometry the cells under investigation experience high pressure and significant shear forces [60]. Therefore a significant number of high Ca^{2+} cells that are more fragile may lyse in the flow cytometer and hence are excluded from the detection.

Furthermore it is worthwhile to mention that under in vivo conditions, cells with a permanent high Ca^{2+} content and/or PS exposure are removed from the circulation, mostly in the spleen, while after long in vitro incubation time (48 h), old RBCs responded with higher increase of intracellular Ca^{2+} content as well as higher PS exposure compared to young RBCs [48, 49].

The intracellular Ca^{2+} content and the PS exposure at the outer membrane leaflet have been investigated for human RBCs also in physiological solutions prepared with oxygen-enriched water (in comparison to normal physiological solution). This was a study for a company (futomat®) producing equipment for the production of oxygen-enriched water for drinking. It has been found that Ca^{2+} content and the PS exposure are not changed significantly in oxygen-enriched water. However, one interesting effect was found when the RBCs were treated with LPA. Under such conditions the PS exposure was significantly reduced in futomat® water compared to normal physiological solution. It remains open and requires clinical studies to see whether there is a relevant effect in human beings, meaning a positive effect preventing thrombus formation.

4. Active role of RBCs in blood coagulation

When the endothelium of blood vessels is damaged, platelets become activated and transport PS to their external membrane surface [50]. After activation, the exposed PS provides a catalytic surface for the formation of active enzyme-substrate complexes of the coagulation cascade, especially for the tenase and prothrombinase complexes [51]. Under these circumstances exposed PS provides a procoagulant surface and is, in general, needed as a response to injury. Therefore, the mechanism of PS exposure has to occur with a relative high transport rate of the lipids. Platelets treated with a Ca^{2+} ionophore show a phospholipid scrambling rate of 78 × 10^3 per second [51]. Human RBCs also show the mechanism of PS exposure after increased intracellular Ca^{2+} content (see above) and are able to adhere to endothelial cells under pathophysiological conditions [22, 52–54]. In addition, exposed PS is sought to serve as a signalling component for macrophages to eliminate old or damaged RBCs from the circulation [55–58]. Since PS-exposing RBCs can adhere to the vascular wall, which may lead to disturbance of the microcirculation [59], the elimination of these cells is a very important mechanism. However, compared to platelets, RBCs have a lower phospholipid scrambling rate (0.45 × 10^3 per second) [51].

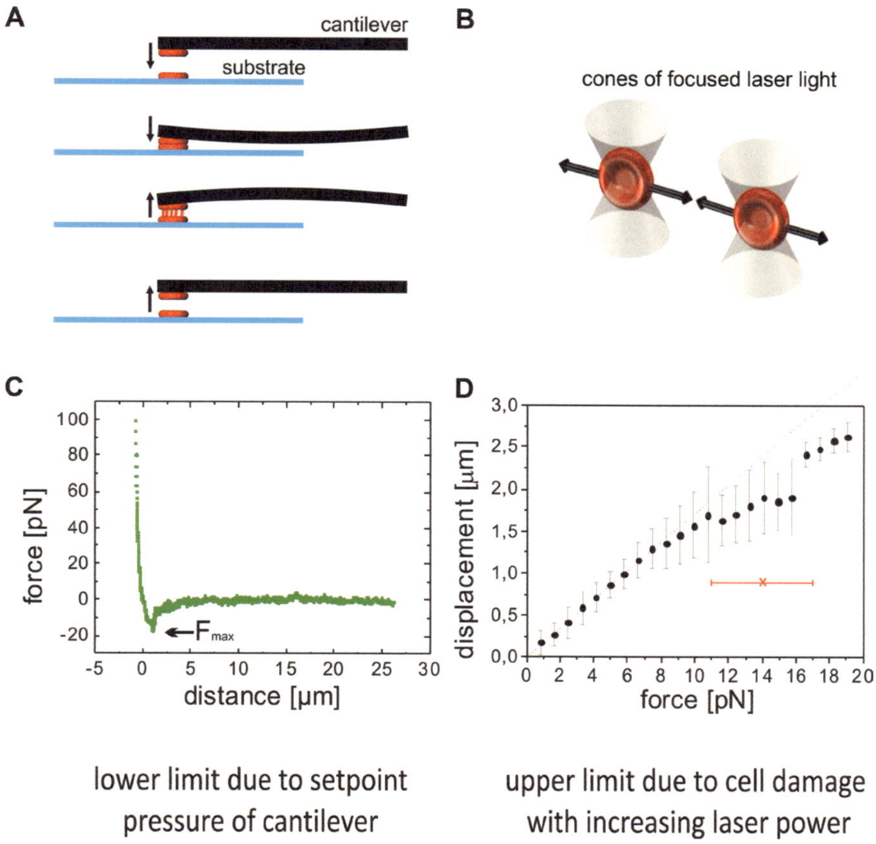

Figure 6.
(A) shows a sketch of the working principle of single-cell force spectroscopy (SCFS). A cell is bound to a cantilever and is brought into contact with another cell at the surface. During the approach and withdrawal of the cell, the deflection is monitored and gives direct information about the adhesion force between the cells. (B) shows a sketch of the working principle of the optical tweezer measurements. Two RBCs are trapped in the foci of two laser beams and are brought into contact. By measuring the deflection of the cells out of the centre of the laser foci, one can determine the adhesion force between the cells. (C) shows a force vs. distance curve derived from the SSFS measurements. A weak interaction of approximately 20 pN can be observed that is mainly due to an artefact of the measurement (see original paper). This 20 pN is the lower limit that one can measure using this type of cell with this technique. (D) shows a force calibration of one RBC in an optical trap. It can be observed that with the given laser power, the trap is only linear up to forces of 15 pN, i.e. this is the upper limit that can be measured with this technique on these types of cells. This figure is reproduced with kind permission from Elsevier. (A) is a reprint from [23], panels (B) and (D) are reprints from [35] and panel (C) is a reprint from [60].

Even more important was the demonstration that human RBCs play an active role in clot formation [23]. This is lacking in medical textbooks, where one can find statements claiming that RBCs only become part of clots because they are so abundant in the circulation. First demonstration of increased interacting forces between two RBCs when the intracellular free Ca^{2+} concentration is increased was performed using non-invasive holographic optical tweezers [23]. In addition, using single-cell force spectroscopy, it has been shown that the upper force limit for Ca^{2+}-triggered adhesion of the RBCs was approximately 100 pN, a value large enough to be of significance during clot formation or in pathological situations [23]. **Figure 6** summarises the in vitro force measurements performed.

5. Active participation of RBCs in thrombotic events

There are numerous indications for the active participation of RBCs in the induction of thrombotic events. The first example we like to mention is the occurrence of thrombotic complications in anaemic patients that experienced a splenectomy. Numerous hereditary anaemic disorders such as spherocytosis, stomatocytosis or elliptocytosis are associated with distorted RBCs, which are preferentially removed in the spleen. Therefore, splenectomy is believed to improve the anaemic symptoms because cells cannot be removed in the spleen. In principle, this concept works out but with the severe side effect that some patients suffer from thrombotic events. Since the 'maintenance' of the RBCs in the spleen is missing, it is likely that the RBCs are the major cause for the thrombotic events. In patients diagnosed with hereditary xerocytosis, mostly related to mutations in the Piezo1 channel, thrombotic complications were regularly reported after these patients underwent splenectomy [61], whereas patients diagnosed for 'Gardos Channelopathy', even after splenectomy, thrombotic events were not observed [62].

An even more prominent example is sickle cell disease associated with vaso-occlusive pain crisis as the major and most severe symptom of the patients. Since the mutation associated with sickle cell disease is in the haemoglobin, it seems obvious that also the symptoms of the disease are associated with RBCs. The common belief is that vaso-occlusive pain crises in sickle cell disease patients are caused by the crystallisation of the mutated haemoglobin under deoxygenation conditions. While the sickle formation under deoxygenation at stasis is undoubted, it's not clear if the same shape change happens in vivo. However, although it is clear that deoxygenated RBCs of sickle cell disease patients have an impaired deformability, the link to the vaso-occlusive crises must be a bit more complicated because deoxygenation happens continuously as deoxygenated RBCs are continuously passing the circulation and vaso-occlusive pain crises happen only sporadically and are so far unpredictable. A possible explanation is the activity of the NMDA-receptors (see above) that are activated by homocysteine and homocysteic acid, which are markers for inflammation in the blood plasma [63].

Such the above described mechanisms triggered by intracellular Ca^{2+} increase are likely to happen also during vaso-occlusive crises in sickle cell disease patients. A first clinical pilot study on sickle cell disease patients using memantine, a drug blocking the NMDA-receptor (and approved to treat Alzheimer disease), showed very promising results both in the support of the mechanism we sketch and in the patients showing a lower number and less severe vaso-occlusive pain crises [64, 65].

Furthermore, it is well known that in RBCs of sickle cell disease patients, the Gardos channel activity is increased [66], which is an indicator for an increased Ca^{2+} since the Gardos channel is a Ca^{2+}-activated K^+ channel. However, a clinical trial testing senicapoc, a Gardos channel inhibitor, failed because vaso-occlusive crises were not improved [66]. Since senicapoc addresses the Gardos channel and not the upstream increase in Ca^{2+} that causes all the effects described above, the failure of senicapoc is explainable.

Additionally, we like to mention and discuss another aspect: The process we describe, in particular the Ca^{2+}-triggered aggregation to initiate thrombus formation, takes some time [23], and an argument is that the time required is too long that aggregation happens between the fast-moving RBCs in the circulation. In this context, we like to mention the hydrodynamic clustering [67], which is perfectly reversible but provides the cellular interaction time since the lifetime of the hydrodynamic clusters can be in the range of several seconds.

6. Conclusions and outlook

It seems obvious that RBC participation in blood coagulation and thrombus formation is more than an accidental trapping in the process. In this chapter we summarised indications, evidences and proofs for active participation of RBCs in blood clotting and thrombus formation. However, this concept so far did not make it into haematological text books and standard medical education. With this book chapter, we like to make a little contribution to better explain and propagate this concept. Although we face severe experimental and clinical evidence for the active participation of RBCs in blood coagulation and thrombus formation, there is a demand for further research on the regulation and manipulation of this aspect in the coagulation sometimes also referred to as RBC hypercoagulation. We are looking forward to the next years of investigations in coagulation and thrombosis research.

Conflict of interest

The authors don't declare a conflict of interests.

Author details

Ingolf Bernhardt*, Mauro C. Wesseling, Duc Bach Nguyen and Lars Kaestner
Saarland University, Saarbrücken, Germany

*Address all correspondence to: i.bernhardt@mx.uni-saarland.de

References

[1] Haest CWM. Distribution and movement of membrane lipids. In: Bernhardt I, Ellory JC, editors. Red Cell Membrane Transport in Health and Disease. Berlin: Springer; 2003. pp. 1-25

[2] Verkleij AJ, Zwaal RFA, Roelofsen B, Comfurius P, Kastelijn D, Van Deenen LLM. The asymmetric distribution of phospholipids in the human red cell membrane. A combined study using phospholipases and freeze-etch electron microscopy. Biochimica et Biophysica Acta. 1973;**323**:178-193

[3] Zwaal RF, Comfurius P, Bevers EM. Surface exposure of phosphatidylserine in pathological cells. Cellular and Molecular Life Sciences. 2005;**62**:971-988

[4] Devaux PF, Herrmann A, Ohlwein N, Kozlov MM. How lipid flippases can modulate membrane structure. Biochimica et Biophysica Acta. 2008;**1778**:1591-1600

[5] Bevers EM, Comfurius P, Dekkers DW, Zwaal RF. Lipid translocation across the plasma membrane of mammalian cells. Biochimica et Biophysica Acta. 1999;**1439**:317-330

[6] Daleke DL. Regulation of phospholipid asymmetry in the erythrocyte membrane. Current Opinion in Hematology. 2008;**15**:191-195

[7] Perez C, Gerber S, Boilevin J, Bucher M, Darbre T, Aebi M, et al. Structure and mechanism of an active lipid-linked oligosaccharide flippase. Nature. 2015;**542**:433-438

[8] Williamson P, Kulick A, Zachowski A, Schlegel RA, Devaux PF. Ca^{2+} induces transbilayer redistribution of all major phospholipids in human erythrocytes. The Biochemist. 1992;**31**:6355-6360

[9] Brunner JD, Lim NK, Schenck S, Duerst A, Dutzler R. X-ray structure of a calcium-activated TMEM16 lipid scramblase. Nature. 2014;**516**:207-212

[10] Lang F, Gulbins E, Lerche H, Huber SM, Kempe DS, Foller M. Eryptosis, a window to systemic disease. Cellular Physiology and Biochemistry. 2008;**22**:373-380

[11] Lang F, Lang KS, Lang PA, Huber SM, Wieder T. Mechanisms and significance of eryptosis. Antioxidants & Redox Signaling. 2006;**8**:1183-1192

[12] Galluzzi L, Vitale I, Aaronson SA, et al. Molecular mechanisms of cell death: Recommendations of the nomenclature committee on cell death. Cell Death and Differentiation. 2018;**25**(3):486-541

[13] Hellem AJ, Borchgrevink CF, Ames SB. The role of red cells in haemostasis: The relation between haematocrit, bleeding time and platelet adhesiveness. British Journal of Haematology. 1961;**7**:42-50

[14] Andrews DA, Low PS. Role of red blood cells in thrombosis. Current Opinion in Hematology. 1999;**6**:76-82

[15] Kaestner L, Christophersen P, Bernhardt I, Bennekou P. The non-selective voltage-activated cation channel in the human red blood cell membrane: Reconciliation between two conflicting reports and further characterisation. Bioelectrochemistry. 2000;**52**:117-125

[16] Kaestner L, Bernhardt I. Ion channels in the human red blood cell membrane: Their further investigation and physiological relevance. Bioelectrochemistry. 2002;**55**:71-74

[17] Kaestner L, Tabellion W, Lipp P, Bernhardt I. Prostaglandin E_2 activates channel-mediated calcium entry in

human erythrocytes: An indication for a blood clot formation supporting process. Thrombosis and Haemostasis. 2004;**92**:1269-1272

[18] Wagner-Britz L, Wang J, Kaestner L, Bernhardt I. Protein kinase Cα and P-type Ca^{2+} channel $Ca_V2.1$ in red blood cell calcium signalling. Cellular Physiology and Biochemistry. 2013;**31**:883-891

[19] Kaestner L. Calcium Signalling: Approaches and Findings in the Heart and Blood. Heidelberg, Berlin, New York: Springer; 2013

[20] Dyrda A, Cytlak U, Ciuraszkiewicz A, Lipinska A, Cueff A, Bouyer G, et al. Local membrane deformations activate Ca^{2+}-dependent K^+ and anionic currents in intact human red blood cells. PLoS One. 2010;**5**:e9447

[21] Kaestner L, Egee S. Commentary: Voltage gating of mechanosensitive PIEZO channels. Frontiers in Physiology. 2018;**9**:1565

[22] Chung SM, Bae ON, Lim KM, Noh JY, Lee MY, Jung YS, et al. Lysophosphatidic acid induces thrombogenic activity through phosphatidylserine exposure and procoagulant microvesicle generation in human erythrocytes. Arteriosclerosis, Thrombosis, and Vascular Biology. 2007;**27**:414-421

[23] Steffen P, Jung A, Nguyen DB, Mueller T, Bernhardt I, Kaestner L, et al. Stimulation of human red blood cell leads to Ca^{2+}-mediated intracellular adhesion. Cell Calcium. 2011;**50**:54-61

[24] Woon LA, Holland JW, Kable EP, Roufogalis BD. Ca^{2+} sensitivity of phospholipid scrambling in human red cell ghosts. Cell Calcium. 1999;**25**:313-320

[25] De Jong K, Rettig MP, Low PS, Kuypers FA. Protein kinase C activation induces phosphatidylserine exposure on red blood cells. Biochemistry. 2002;**41**:12562-12567

[26] Klarl BA, Lang PA, Kempe DS, Niemoeller OM, Akel A, Sobiesiak M, et al. Protein kinase C mediates erythrocyte "programmed cell death" following glucose depletion. American Journal of Physiology. Cell Physiology. 2006;**290**:C244-C253

[27] Nelson GJ. Lipid composition of erythrocytes in various mammalian species. Biochimica et Biophysica Acta. 1967;**144**(2):221-232

[28] Nouri-Sorkhabi MH, Agar NS, Sullivan DR, Gallagher C, Kuchel PW. Phospholipid composition of erythrocyte membranes and plasma of mammalian blood including Australian marsupials; quantitative 31P NMR analysis using detergent. Comparative Biochemistry and Physiology. 1996;**113B**:221-227

[29] Oonishi T, Sakashita K, Ishioka N, Suematsu N, Shio H, Uyesaka N. Production of prostaglandins E_1 and E_2 by adult human red blood cells. Prostaglandins & Other Lipid Mediators. 1998;**56**:89-101

[30] Nguyen DB, Wagner-Britz L, Maia S, Steffen P, Wagner C, Kaestner L, et al. Regulation of phosphatidylserine exposure in red blood cells. Cellular Physiology and Biochemistry. 2011;**28**:847-856

[31] Wang J, Wagner-Britz L, Bogdanova A, Ruppenthal S, Wiesen K, Kaiser E, et al. Morphologically homogeneous red blood cells present a heterogeneous response to hormonal stimulation. PLoS One. 2013;**8**(6):e67697

[32] Yang L, Andrews DA, Low PS. Lysophosphatidic acid opens a Ca(++) channel in human erythrocytes. Blood. 2000;**95**(7):2420-2425

[33] Andrews DA, Yang LPS. Phorbol ester stimulates a protein kinase C-mediated agatoxin-TK-sensitive

calcium permeability pathway in human red blood cells. Blood. 2002;**100**(9):3392-3399

[34] Wesseling MC, Wagner-Britz L, Nguyen DB, Asanidze S, Mutua J, Mohamed N, et al. Novel insights in the regulation of phosphatidylserine exposure in human red blood cells. Cellular Physiology and Biochemistry. 2016;**39**:1941-1954

[35] Kaestner L, Steffen P, Nguyen DB, Wang J, Wagner-Britz L, Jung A, et al. Lysophosphatidic acid induced red blood cell aggregation in vitro. Bioelectrochemistry. 2012;**87**:89-95

[36] Kaestner L, Bogdanova A, Egee S. Calcium channels and calcium-regulated channels in human red blood cells. In: Islam S, editor. Calcium Signalling. Berlin, Heidelberg, New York: Springer; 2019. In press

[37] Makhro A, Wang J, Vogel J, Boldyrev AA, Gassmann M, Kaestner L, et al. Functional NMDA receptors in mammalian erythrocytes. American Journal of Physiology-Cell Physiology. 2010;**298**:C1315-C1325

[38] Makhro A, Hanggi P, Goede J, Wang J, Bruggemann A, Gassmann M, et al. N-Methyl D-aspartate (NMDA) receptors in human erythroid precursor cells and in circulating red blood cells contribute to the intracellular calcium regulation. American Journal of Physiology-Cell Physiology. 2013;**305**:C1123-C1138

[39] Sibarov DA, Giniatullin R, Antonov SM. High sensitivity of cerebellar neurons to homocysteine is determined by expression of GluN2C and GluN2D subunits of NMDA receptors. Biochemical and Biophysical Research Communications. 2018;**506**:648-652

[40] Hertz L, Huisjes R, Llaudet-Planas E, Petkova-Kirova P, Makhro A, Danielczok J, et al. Is increased intracellular calcium in red blood cells a common component in the molecular mechanism causing anemia? Frontiers in Physiology. 2017;**8**:673

[41] Lang KS, Lang PA, Bauer C, Duranton C, Wieder T, Huber SM, et al. Mechanisms of suicidal erythrocyte death. Cellular Physiology and Biochemistry. 2005;**15**:195-202

[42] Foeller M, Huber SM, Lang F. Erythrocyte programmed cell death. IUBMB Life. 2008;**60**:661-668

[43] Anderson DR, Davis JL, Carraway KL. Calcium-promoted changes of the human erythrocyte membrane. Involvement of spectrin, transglutaminase, and a membrane-bound protease. The Journal of Biological Chemistry. 1977;**252**:6617-6623

[44] Hatanaka M, Yoshimura N, Murakami T, Kannagi R, Murachi T. Evidence for membrane-associated calpain I in human erythrocytes. Detection by an immunoelectrophoretic blotting method using monospecific antibody. The Biochemist. 1984;**23**:3272-3276

[45] Lofvenberg L, Backman L. Calpain-induced proteolysis of beta-spectrins. FEBS Letters. 1999;**443**:89-92

[46] Choi JW, Herr DR, Noguchi K, Yung YC, Lee C, Mutoh T, et al. LPA receptors: Subtypes and biological actions. Annual Review of Pharmacology and Toxicology. 2010;**50**:157-186

[47] Lutz HU, Stammler P, Fasler S, Ingold M, Fehr J. Density separation of human red blood cells on self-forming Percoll gradients: Correlation with age. Biochimica et Biophysica Acta. 1992;**1116**:1-10

[48] Wesseling MC, Wagner-Britz L, Huppert H, Hanf B, Hertz L, Nguyen

DB, et al. Phosphatidylserine exposure in human red blood cells depending on cell age. Cellular Physiology and Biochemistry. 2016;**38**:1376-1390

[49] Ghashghaeinia M, Cluitmans JC, Akel A, Dreischer D, Toulany M, Köberle M, et al. The impact of erythrocyte age on eryptosis. British Journal of Haematology. 2012;**157**:606-614

[50] Heemskerk JW, Bevers EM, Lindhout T. Platelet activation and blood coagulation. Thrombosis and Haemostasis. 2002;**88**:186-193

[51] Williamson P, Christie A, Kohlin T, Schlegel RA, Comfurius P, Harmsma M, et al. Phospholipid scramblase activation pathways in lymphocytes. The Biochemist. 2001;**40**:8065-8072

[52] Betal SG, Setty YB. Phosphatidylserine-positive erythrocytes bind to immobilized and soluble thrombospndin-1 via its heparin binding domain. Translational Research. 2008;**152**:165-177

[53] Closse C, Dachary-Progent J, Boisseau MR. Phosphatidylserine-related adhesion of human erythrocytes to vascular endothelium. British Journal of Haematology. 1999;**107**:300-302

[54] Gallagher PG, Chang SH, Rettig MP, Neely JE, Hillery CA, Smith BD, et al. Altered erythrocyte endothelial adherence and membrane phospholipid asymmetry in hereditary hydrocytosis. Blood. 2003;**101**:4625-4627

[55] Boas FE, Forman L, Beutler E. Phosphatidylserine exposure and red cell viability in red cell aging and in hemolytic anemia. Proceedings of the National Academy of Sciences of the United States of America. 1998;**95**:3077-3081

[56] Fadok VA, Bratton DL, Rose DM, Pearson A, Ezekewitz RA, Henson PM. A receptor for phosphatidylserine-specific clearance of apoptotic cells. Nature. 2000;**405**:85-90

[57] McEvoy L, Williamson P, Schlegel RA. Membrane phospholipid asymmetry as a determinant of erythrocyte recognition by macrophages. Proceedings of the National Academy of Sciences of the United States of America. 1986;**83**:3311-3315

[58] Schroit AJ, Madsen JW, Tanaka Y. *In vivo* recognition and clearance of red blood cells containing phosphatidylserine in their plasma membranes. The Journal of Biological Chemistry. 1985;**260**:5131-5138

[59] Bouguerra G, Aljanadi O, Bissinger R, Abbès S, Lang F. Embelin-induced phosphatidylserine translocation in the erythrocyte cell membrane. Cellular Physiology and Biochemistry. 2015;**37**:1629-1640

[60] Minetti G, Egee S, Mörsdorf D, Steffen P, Makhro A, Achilli C, et al. Red cell investigations: Art and artefacts. Blood Reviews. 2013;**27**:91-101

[61] Stewart GW, Amess JA, Eber SW, Kingswood C, Lane PA, Smith BD, et al. Thrombo-embolic disease after splenectomy for hereditary stomatocytosis. British Journal of Haematology. 1996;**93**:303-310

[62] Fermo E, Bogdanova AY, Petkova-Kirova P, Zaninoni A, Marcello AP, Makhro A, et al. 'Gardos Channelopathy': A variant of hereditary stomatocytosis with complex molecular regulation. Scientific Reports. 2017;**7**:1744

[63] Wu JT. Circulating homocysteine is an inflammation marker and a risk factor of life-threatening inflammatory diseases. Journal of Biomedical and Laboratory Sciences. 2007;**19**(4):107-111

[64] Hegemann I, Sasselli C, Valeri F, Makhro A, Müller R, Bogdanova A, et al. Memantine Treatment is Well Tolerated by Sickle Cell Patients and Improves Erythrocyte Stability: Phase II Study MemSID; 2019

[65] Bogdanova A, Makhro A, Hegemann I, Seiler E, Bogdanov N, Simionato G, Kaestner L, et al. Improved Maturation and Increased Stability of Red Blood Cells of Sickle Cell Patients on Memantine Treatment; 2019

[66] Ataga KI, Reid M, Ballas SK, Yasin Z, Bigelow C, James LS, et al. Improvements in haemolysis and indicators of erythrocyte survival do not correlate with acute vaso-occlusive crises in patients with sickle cell disease: A phase III randomized, placebo-controlled, double-blind study of the Gardos channel blocker senicapoc (ICA-17043). British Journal of Haematology. 2011;**153**:92-104

[67] Brust M, Aouane O, Thiébaud M, Flormann D, Verdier C, Kaestner L, et al. The plasma protein fibrinogen stabilizes clusters of red blood cells in microcapillary flows. Scientific Reports. 2014;**4**:4348

Chapter 4

Who Is Balancing: Is It RBC or Acid-Base Status?

T. Rajini Samuel

Abstract

Hemoglobin is an important intracellular protein buffer present inside the red blood cells (RBC). When the partial pressure of carbon dioxide (pCO_2) is increased, it freely diffuses into the RBC where it reacts with water molecules to form carbonic acid which dissociates to form bicarbonate and hydrogen ions by the enzyme carbonic anhydrase. Hydrogen ions liberated in this reaction are buffered by hemoglobin. Oxyhemoglobin is a stronger acid than deoxyhemoglobin. Oxygenation of hemoglobin causes an increase in net titratable hydrogen ion due to the Haldane effect. As the oxygen saturation of hemoglobin (sO_2) increases, the base excess is changed in the acidic direction, or as the sO_2 decreases, the base excess is changed in alkaline direction. The changes in the level of the enzyme carbonic anhydrase in RBC are related to the changes in pH, pCO_2, and bicarbonate levels in the blood. The understanding of the acid-base balance is a challenging task, but at the same time, it has immense clinical value. The relationship of carbonic anhydrase enzyme present inside the RBC in maintaining the acid-base balance to the commonly employed arterial blood gas (ABG) parameters like pH, pCO_2 bicarbonate, and base excess may help us for better understanding.

Keywords: acid-base balance, carbonic anhydrase enzyme, oxygen saturation, hemoglobin

1. Introduction

Arterial blood gas (ABG) analysis plays a vital role in the management of intensive care unit patients, especially for critically ill patients, but the interpretation is sometimes a challenging task especially if the acid-base disturbances are complex [1–5]. In ABG analysis, the pH and pCO_2 are measured parameters, but bicarbonate concentration is a calculated parameter derived from the modified Henderson equation [2]. Davenport or bicarbonate-pH diagram is a graphical tool representing the relationship between pH, pCO_2, and bicarbonate to depict the respiratory and metabolic acid-base disturbances. This Davenport diagram is rarely used in clinical setting [1].

Simple acid-base disorders are very easy to diagnose, but combined acid-base disorders due to either *compensatory* mechanisms or *mixed disorders* are often difficult and sometimes confusing. The *four acid-base disorders* are metabolic acidosis, metabolic alkalosis, respiratory acidosis, and respiratory alkalosis. Simple acid-base disorder is the presence of any of the four disorders with appropriate compensations. *Mixed acid-base disorder* denotes the presence of more than one primary disturbances which can be suspected from a lesser or greater than expected compensations. *Respiratory disorders* are associated with appropriate renal compensatory mechanisms, and similarly metabolic disorders are compensated by respiratory mechanisms [6, 7].

Base excess is defined as the amount of strong acid that must be added to each liter of fully oxygenated blood to return the pH to 7.40 at a temperature of 37°C and a pCO_2 of 40 mmHg. The normal level for base excess is −2 to +2 mEq/L. A negative base excess indicates the presence of base deficit. Actual base excess is the base excess of the blood, while standard base excess is the base excess of the *extracellular fluid (ECF)* at hemoglobin concentration of 5 gm/dL [8–10].

Under *normal ventilation*, bicarbonate parameter is useful, but in patients with abnormal ventilation (respiration), it may not reflect the true status because bicarbonate is a dependent variable and it changes with the concentration of pCO_2. As pCO_2 increases, it reacts with *water molecules* to form *carbonic acid* which dissociates into *hydrogen* and *bicarbonate* ions. The hydrogen ions are buffered by *non-bicarbonate buffers* like albumin, hemoglobin, and phosphate buffer system. So, the concentration of bicarbonate increases as pCO_2 also increases. This *problem is solved by* measuring standard bicarbonate [11, 12].

Standard bicarbonate is the concentration of bicarbonate in the plasma from blood which is equilibrated with a normal pCO_2 (40 mmHg) and a normal pO_2 (over 100 mmHg) at a normal temperature (37°C). The *actual bicarbonate* and the *standard bicarbonate* concentrations are approximately equal under normal ventilation, but in abnormal respiration (either hypoventilation or hyperventilation), the two values alter and deviate from each other depending on the changes in the concentration of pCO_2 [1].

The bicarbonate value is increased in respiratory acidosis and decreased in respiratory alkalosis. So, the difference between bicarbonate and standard bicarbonate value is positive for respiratory acidosis and negative for respiratory alkalosis. If the acid-base disorder is purely metabolic without respiratory compensation, then the bicarbonate and standard bicarbonate values are more or less closer. If the metabolic disorder is compensated by respiratory mechanisms, then the two values alter and deviate from each other.

The most commonly used approach for arterial blood gas (ABG) analysis interpretation is a physiological approach based on the bicarbonate-carbon dioxide buffer system. The major buffer system in the ECF is the carbon dioxide-bicarbonate buffer system, and other buffer systems that play a role in buffering are protein and phosphate buffer systems. The buffers are substances that resist changes in pH. All buffers in a common solution are in equilibrium with the same hydrogen ion concentration. Therefore, whenever there is a change in hydrogen ion concentration in the extracellular fluid, the balance of all the buffer systems changes at the same time. This phenomenon is called the isohydric principle. Henderson-Hasselbalch equation concentrating on the bicarbonate-pCO_2 buffer is based on this principle. This approach is very simple and easier, but a major drawback of this is it is unable to quantify the metabolic (non-respiratory) component and does not explain the causative mechanism of metabolic acid-base disturbances [8].

2. Base excess

Base excess approach was developed to quantify the metabolic component, but it was *criticized* because it represents the whole blood and *did not* accurately *represent* the *whole body behavior*. Blood volume diluted with interstitial fluid represents the effective extracellular fluid hemoglobin concentration of 5 g/dl. *Standard base excess* or extracellular base excess is the base excess at hemoglobin concentration of 5 g/dl [8–12].

Oxyhemoglobin is a stronger acid than deoxyhemoglobin. Oxygenation of hemoglobin causes an increase in net titratable hydrogen ion because hydrogen ions are liberated from the oxygen-linked buffer groups due to the Haldane effect. So, the variation of oxygen saturation of hemoglobin (sO_2) influences the base excess result. The formula for calculating this is

$$\text{cBase}(\text{B, oxygenated}) = \text{cBase}(\text{B, actual}) - 0.2 \times \text{ctHb} \times (1 - \text{sO}_2)$$

or

$$cBase(B, actual) = cBase(B, oxygenated) + 0.2 \times ctHb \times (1 - sO_2)$$

As the sO_2 increases, the term $0.2 \times \text{ctHb} \times (1 - \text{sO}_2)$ decreases, so the base excess is changed in the acidotic direction because it is slightly decreased, or as the sO_2 decreases, the term $0.2 \times \text{ctHb} \times (1 - \text{sO}_2)$ increases, so the base excess is changed in alkaline direction because it is slightly increased [8–10].

The correlation between pCO_2 and (HCO_3 − standard HCO_3)/H_2CO_3 and pCO_2 and ratio of (HCO_3/standard HCO_3) is clearly shown in **Figures 1** and **2**, respectively. From that, it is very clear that as the pCO_2 decreases, the ratio of (HCO_3 − standard HCO_3)/H_2CO_3 also decreases and, as the pCO_2 increases, the ratio of (HCO_3 − standard HCO_3)/H_2CO_3 also increases and, thereafter, the curve flattens. At pCO_2 of 40 mmHg, the ratio of (HCO_3 − standard HCO_3)/H_2CO_3 is zero because the difference between bicarbonate and standard bicarbonate value is zero (HCO_3 − standard HCO_3 is zero). In respiratory acidosis (due to hypoventilation), pCO_2 retention occurs, and in respiratory alkalosis (due to hyperventilation), the pCO_2 value is decreased. The ratio of (HCO_3 − standard HCO_3)/H_2CO_3 changes in respiratory disorders and also in metabolic acid-base disturbances associated with respiratory compensations. The ratio of (HCO_3 − standard HCO_3)/H_2CO_3 is greater positive for respiratory acidosis and greater negative for respiratory alkalosis [1].

The normal range for standard base excess is ±2 mmol/L. If the value is >2 mmol/L, then it denotes metabolic alkalosis, and if the value is <−2 mmol/L, then it denotes metabolic acidosis (base deficit). Using this concept a four-quadrant graphical tool can be constructed for ABG interpretation using standard base excess

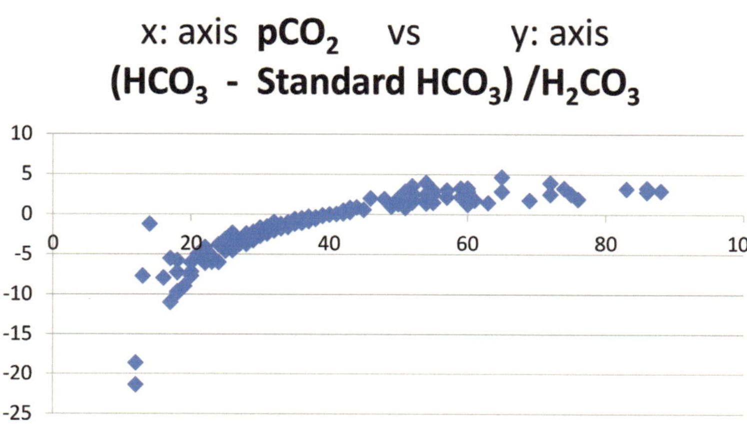

Figure 1.
Relation between pCO_2 and (HCO_3 − standard HCO_3)/H_2CO_3.

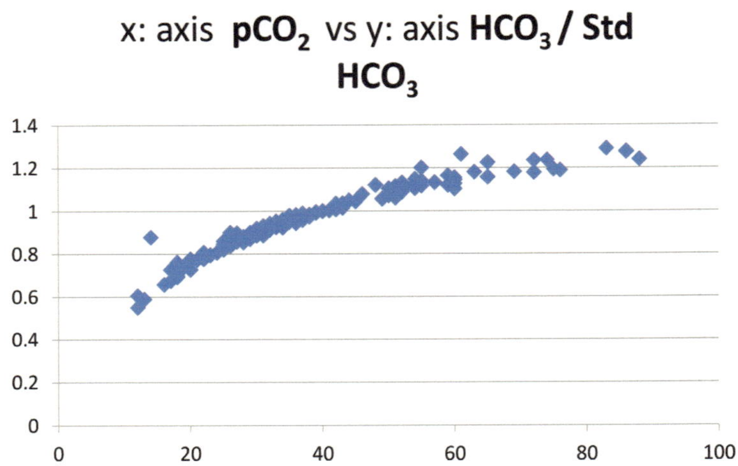

Figure 2.
Relation between pCO_2 *and* $HCO_3/Std\ HCO_3$.

and the ratio of (HCO_3 – standard HCO_3)/H_2CO_3 in the two axes that demarcate the various acid-base disturbances which are shown in **Figure 3** [1].

The aim of the manuscript is to increase in depth the understanding of the acid-base balance which is a challenging and at times an arduous task, yet it has immense

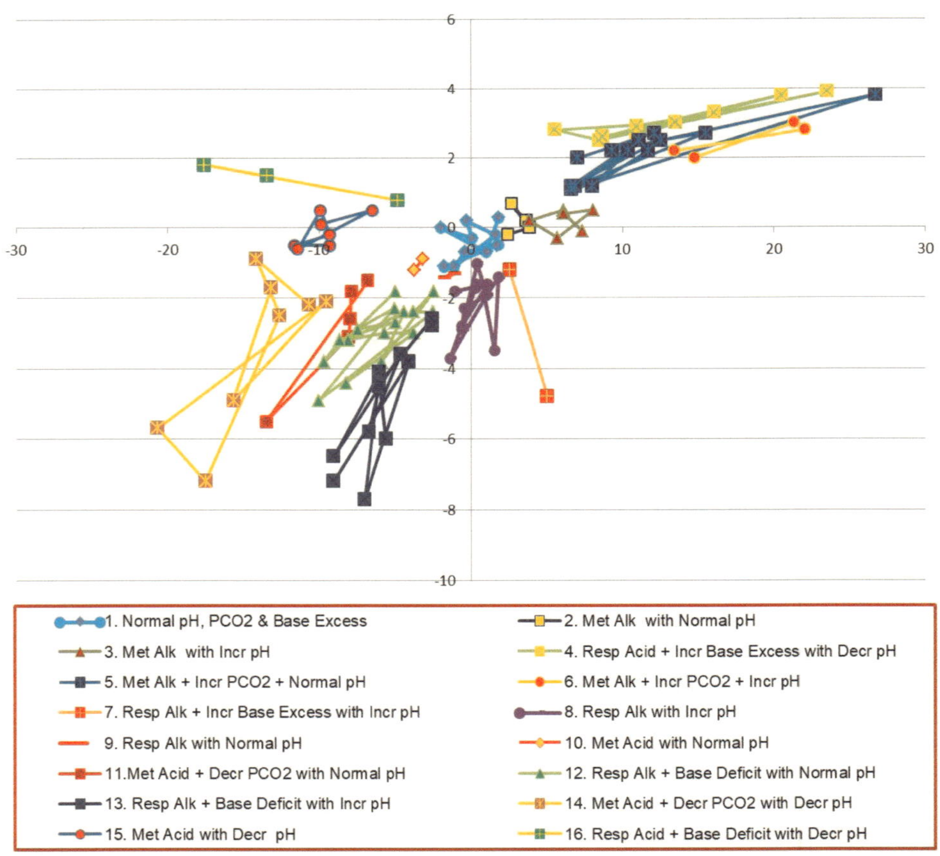

Figure 3.
Analysis of various acid-base disturbances using standard base excess (x-axis) and the ratio of (HCO_3 – *standard* HCO_3)/H_2CO_3 *(y-axis) in the four-quadrant graph.*

clinical value. The relationship of the formation of bicarbonate from pCO_2 with the help of carbonic anhydrase enzyme present inside the RBC plays a significant role in maintaining the acid-base balance. The application of standard bicarbonate in the calculation of non-respiratory hydrogen ion concentration and development of a novel four quadrant graphical method for arterial blood gas interpretation may help us for better understanding.

3. Materials and methods

About 188 arterial blood gas sample data were utilized. Strict precautions were taken to avoid pre-analytical errors, and the consistency of the ABG report was checked by using the modified Henderson equation [2].

The main parameters like measured *pH*, pCO_2, HCO_3, *standard* HCO_3, and *standard base excess* values were noted. *Carbonic acid* concentration was calculated from pCO_2. The difference between bicarbonate and standard bicarbonate was calculated. The ratio of $(HCO_3 - \text{standard } HCO_3)/H_2CO_3$ was calculated [1].

Calculation of H^+:

H^+—hydrogen ion concentration at actual pH
(Calculated using *modified Henderson equation*)

$$H^+ \text{ (hydrogen ion concentration)} = \{24 \times pCO_2\}/HCO_3$$

$$pH = -\log[H^+ \text{ nanomoles/L}]$$
$$= -\log[H^+ \times 10^{-9} \text{ moles/L}]$$
$$= -\log[H^+] - \log[10^{-9}] \; \{\text{nanomoles/L} = 10^{-9} \text{ moles/L}\}$$
$$pH = 9 - \log[H^+]$$

Calculation of NRH^+ *(non-respiratory hydrogen ion concentration):*

NRH^+—hydrogen ion concentration at non-respiratory pH
(At pCO_2 of 40 mmHg)

This calculated hydrogen ion concentration equivalent of standard bicarbonate has thus been called the "non-respiratory" hydrogen ion concentration or NRH^+ [13, 14]. It has a unique value for a given standard bicarbonate concentration, and the relationship is clearly shown in **Figure 4**:

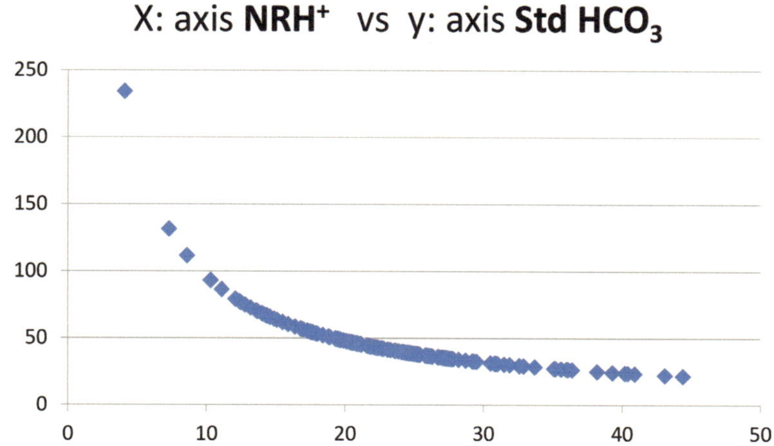

Figure 4.
Relation between NRH^+ *and Std* HCO_3.

$NRH^+ = \{24 \times pCO_2\}/\text{Std } HCO_3$
$= \{24 \times 40\}/\text{Std } HCO_3$ (pCO_2 is *40 mmHg*)
$NRH^+ = 960/\text{Std } HCO_3$
$NRpH = 9 - \log [NRH^+]$

Calculation of ΔRpH:

$pH = 9 - \log [H^+]$
$NRpH = 9 - \log [NRH^+]$
$pH - NRpH = 9 - \log [H^+] - 9 + \log [NRH^+]$
$= \log [NRH^+/H^+]$ or $-\log [H^+/NRH^+]$
H^+ (hydrogen ion concentration) $= \{24 \times pCO_2\}/HCO_3$
NRH^+ (non-respiratory hydrogen ion concentration)
$= \{24 \times 40\}/\text{Std } HCO_3$
$[NRH^+]/[H^+] = \{24 \times 40\}/\text{Std } HCO_3/\{24 \times pCO_2\}/HCO_3$
$= 40 \times \{(HCO_3/\text{Std } HCO_3)/pCO_2\}$
Or in terms of carbonic acid [$pCO_2 = H_2CO_3/0.03$], this can be written as
$= 1.2 \times \{(HCO_3/\text{Std } HCO_3)/H_2CO_3\}$
$pH - NRpH = \log [NRH^+/H^+]$
$pH - NRpH = \log 40 + \log (HCO_3/\text{Std } HCO_3) - \log(pCO_2)$
$[pH - NRpH] = 1.6 + \log\{(HCO_3/\text{Std } HCO_3)/pCO_2\}$

At pCO_2 of *40 mmHg*, *pH − NRpH* is *zero* (because bicarbonate and standard bicarbonate values are equal, log 1 is zero, and log 40 is 1.6). At higher pCO_2 levels (>*40 mmHg*), the value of [*pH − NRpH*] is *negative* which denotes the *acidic influence* of increased pCO_2. At lower pCO_2 levels (<*40 mmHg*), the value of [*pH − NRpH*] is *positive* which denotes the *alkaline influence* of decreased pCO_2:

$[pH - NRpH] = 1.6 + \log \{(HCO_3/\text{Std } HCO_3)/pCO_2\}$
where NRpH denotes the non-respiratory pH.
$pH = 9 - \log [H^+]$
$NRpH = 9 - \log [NRH^+]$
$pH - NRpH = 9 - \log [H^+] - 9 + \log [NRH^+]$
$= \log [NRH^+]/[H^+]$ or $-\log [[H^+]/[NRH^+]$

The *magnitude* and *direction* (positive or negative) of the changes in the parameter *ΔRpH* (pH − NRpH) denote the respiratory influence in causing changes in pH. The value is *negative* for *acidic* effect and *positive* for *alkaline* effect. At pCO_2 of *40 mmHg*, pH − NRpH is *zero* [14].

3.1 Net changes in total pH

The net changes in *total pH* (actual pH) include both the changes in *respiratory* and *non-respiratory* (metabolic) components affecting the pH [14]:

$\Delta pH = \Delta RpH + \Delta NRpH$
$pH - 7.4 = \Delta RpH + NRpH - 7.4$

where ΔNRpH (NRpH − 7.4) denotes the changes in pH due to metabolic component.

3.2 Predicted respiratory pH

$pH = 7.4 + \Delta RpH + \Delta NRpH$
$7.4 + \Delta RpH - pH = -\Delta NRpH$
$Pr\ RpH - pH = -\Delta NRpH$ $\{Pr\ RpH$ (predicted respiratory pH) $= 7.4 + \Delta RpH\}$

The predicted respiratory pH is the *pH* at which the *changes in pH* due to *metabolic* component are *zero* (*ΔNRpH is zero*).

The difference between the *predicted respiratory pH* and *actual pH* denotes the changes in pH due to metabolic component. The *magnitude* and *direction* (positive or negative) of the changes in the parameter *ΔNRpH* (NRpH − 7.4) are due to the accumulation of acids other than carbonic acid or bases. The value is *negative* for *acidic* effect and *positive* for *alkaline* effect. This is one of the postulates of the acid-base balance theory recently published. If the *actual pH* is *less* than the *predicted respiratory pH*, *ΔNRpH* is *negative*. If the *actual pH* is *greater* than the *predicted respiratory pH*, *ΔNRpH* is *positive* [15–18].

NRPH-7.4:

$$NRPH\text{-}7.4 = 9 - \log[NRH^+] - \{9 - \log[40]$$
$$= 9 - \log[NRH^+] - 9 + \log[40]$$
$$= \log\{[40]/[NRH^+]\ \text{or}\ -\log\{[NRH^+]/[40]\}$$

7.4 + ΔRpH:

$$7.4 + \Delta RpH = \{9 - \log[40] + 9 - \log[H^+] - 9 + \log[NRH^+]$$
$$= 9 + \log[NRH^+]/\{[H^+] \times [40]\}$$
$$\{\Delta RpH\ (pH - NRpH) = 9 - \log[H^+] - 9 + \log[NRH^+]\}$$
$$= \log\{[NRH^+]/[H^+]\}\text{or} -\log\{[H^+]/[NRH^+]\}$$

Pr Resp Ph related to $[NRH^+]/\{[H^+] \times [40]\}$

3.3 Net changes in total hydrogen ion concentration

The sum total changes in the hydrogen ion concentration ($\Delta H^+ = [H^+] - [40]$) in the blood include both the changes due to respiratory ($\Delta RH^+ = [H^+] - [NRH^+]$) and non-respiratory (metabolic) components ($\Delta NRH^+ = [NRH^+] - [40]$):

$$[\Delta RH^+/H^+] = [H^+ - NRH^+]/[H^+] = 1 - \{[NRH^+]/[H^+]\}$$
$$[\Delta NRH^+/40] = (NRH^+ - 40)/40\ \text{or}$$
$$-[\Delta NRH^+/40] = (40 - NRH^+)/40$$
$$= 1 - \{(NRH^+/40)\}.$$

The hydrogen ion concentration is 40 at *pH 7.4* which denotes the *homeostatic set point* of acid-base balance [14, 18].

4. New graphical tool

This new graphical tool developed for ABG interpretation contains four quadrants. In the x-axis, standard base excess values were taken, and in the y-axis, the ratio of (HCO_3 − standard HCO_3)/H_2CO_3 values was taken to analyze the various acid-base disturbances which are clearly shown in the four-quadrant graph (**Figure 3**).

In the *first quadrant* (both x- and y-axes are positive), if the plotted area is toward the x-axis, then it represents metabolic alkalosis, and if the area is toward the y-axis, then it represents respiratory acidosis. The plotted area in between and higher may represent combined acid-base disturbances (metabolic alkalosis and respiratory acidosis). The combined acid-base disturbances may be due to compensatory mechanism or mixed acid-base disorders.

In the *second quadrant* (the x-axis is positive, and the y-axis negative), if the plotted area is toward the y-axis, then it represents respiratory alkalosis, and if the area is in between and lower, then it may represent combined acid-base disturbances (metabolic alkalosis and respiratory alkalosis).

In the *third quadrant* (both x- and y-axes are negative), if the plotted area is toward the x-axis, then it represents metabolic acidosis, and if the area is in between and lower, then it represents both metabolic acidosis and respiratory alkalosis. In the *fourth quadrant* (the x-axis is negative and the y-axis is positive), if the area is toward the y-axis, then it represents respiratory acidosis, and if the area is in between and higher, then it may represent both metabolic acidosis and respiratory acidosis [1].

The *acid-base disorders* can be classified and plotted in the *four-quadrant graph* by using the values of standard base excess and the ratio of (HCO_3 – standard HCO_3)/H_2CO_3. Each acid-base disorder will occupy any of the four quadrants, and the normal ABG analysis reports will be seen around the center of the graph. ABG interpretation is very essential for critically ill patients. Immediate analysis, interpretation, and prompt treatment may reduce the morbidity and mortality of the patients. [1] This newer graphical tool may provide a rough guide and help in easier and quicker interpretation of ABG reports. A minor drawback of this graphical tool is that, as the pCO_2 increases, the *ratio of (HCO_3 – standard HCO_3)/H_2CO_3* also increases and afterward the curve flattens. This may not clearly demarcate the different higher levels of pCO_2 values. Although the ratio of (HCO_3 – standard HCO_3)/H_2CO_3 differentiates the respiratory acidosis and respiratory alkalosis, it may not clearly differentiate the different pCO_2 levels. But this can be *corrected (rectified)* in a three-dimensional graph if pCO_2 values are included in the third axis (z-axis). The parameter *(pCO_2 – 40 mmHg)* should be taken in the third axis, because the ratio (HCO_3 – standard HCO_3)/H_2CO_3 is zero at *pCO_2 of 40 mmHg*, so that the *zero central point* is *common* to all the three parameters of the three axes [18].

Arterial blood gas reports should be interpreted with clinical correlation. This newer graphical tool clearly demonstrates that the different acid-base disorders in a four-quadrant graph method may provide a rough guide to interpret the results quickly and easily. The current research study tries to emphasize the clinical significance of this newer diagnostic tool, which, used along with other ABG parameters and proper clinical correlation, may help in better interpretation of ABG reports.

The concept of non-respiratory hydrogen ion concentration plays a key role in understanding of ABG interpretation, yet often it is not discussed in detail during

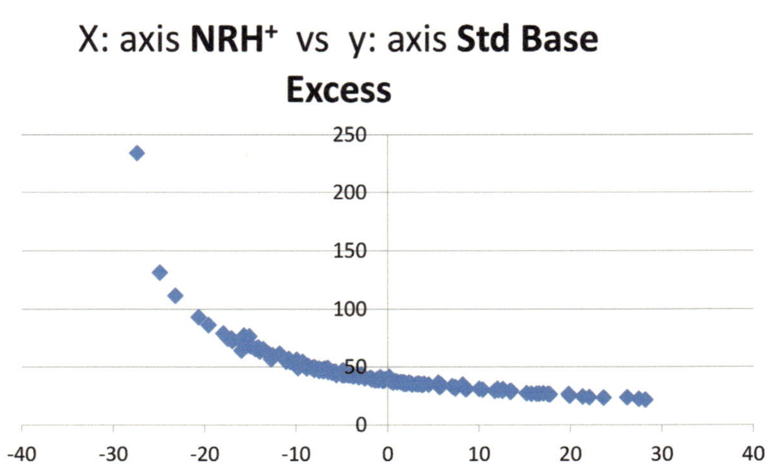

Figure 5.
Relation between NRH^+ and Std base excess.

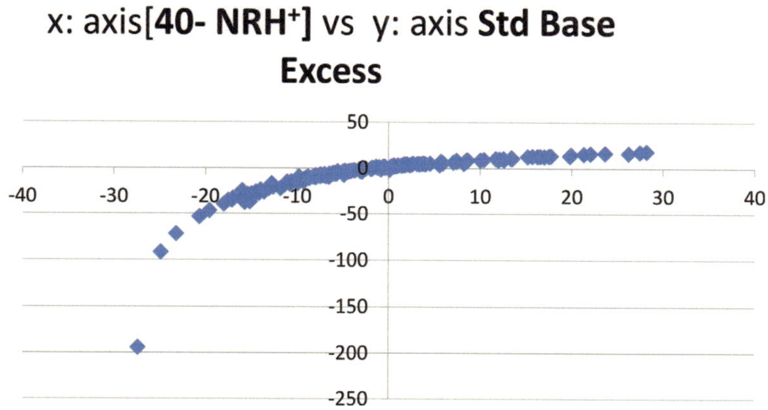

Figure 6.
Relation between [40 − NRH⁺] and Std base excess.

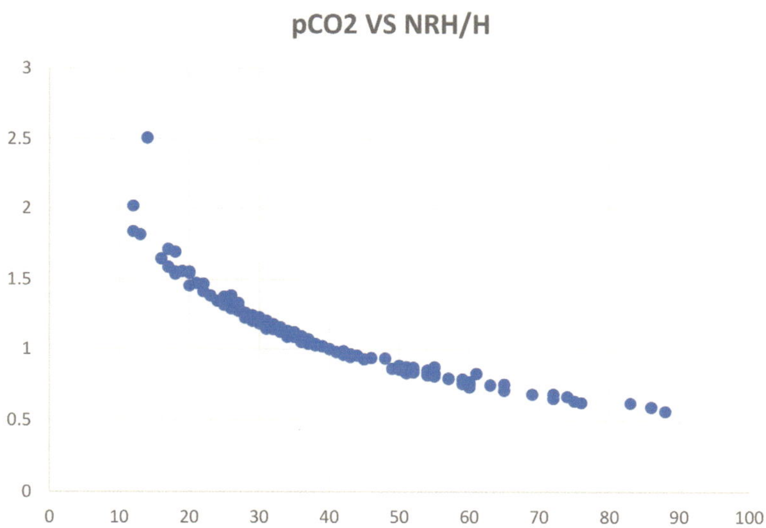

Figure 7.
X-axis pCO_2 vs. y-axis [NRH]/[H].

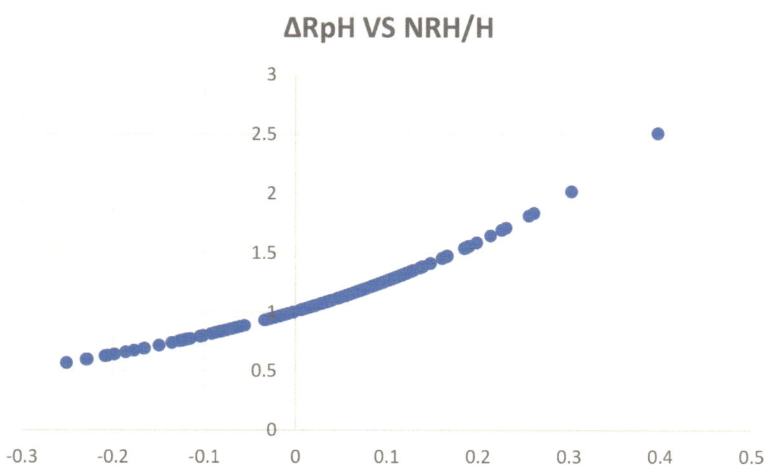

Figure 8.
X-axis ΔRpH vs. y-axis [NRH]/[H].

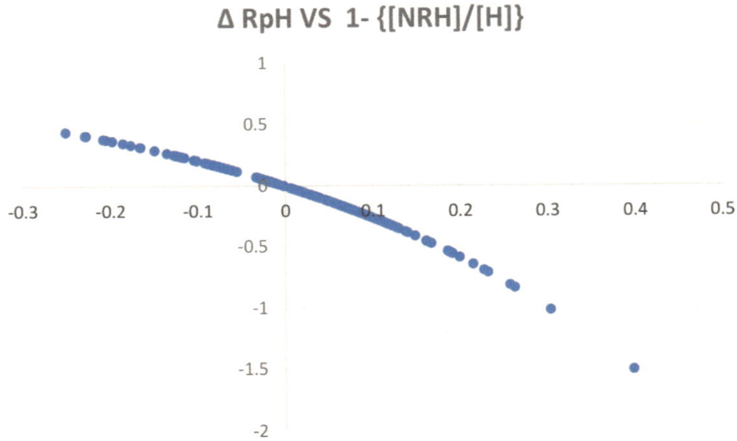

Figure 9.
X-axis ΔRpH vs. y-axis $1 - \{[NRH]/[H]\}$.

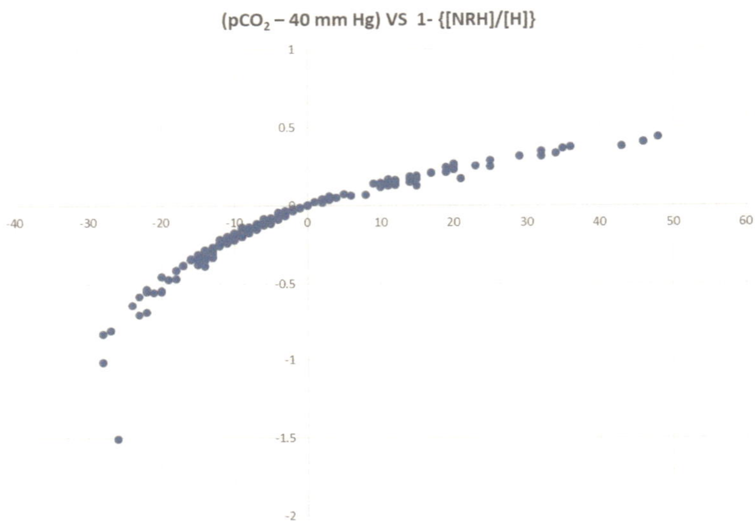

Figure 10.
X-axis $(pCO_2 - 40\ mmHg)$ vs. y-axis $1 - \{[NRH]/[H]\}$.

S. no	pH	pCO_2	HCO_3	Std HCO_3	pH-7.4	ΔRpH	ΔNRpH NRPH-7.4	Pr RpH 7.4 + ΔRpH
1.	7.26	31	13.9	15.5	−0.14	0.06	−0.20	7.46
Comment: changes in *net pH (acidic)* are *mainly* due to *metabolic* component, *partly opposed* by *respiratory* component (*alkaline effect*)								
2.	7.5	37	28.9	29.2	0.1	0.03	0.07	7.43
3.	7.48	43	32	30.9	0.08	−0.02	0.10	7.38
Comment: changes in *net pH (alkaline)* are mainly due to *metabolic* component								
4.	7.41	37	23.5	24.3	0.01	0.02	−0.01	7.42
5.	7.39	38	23	23.6	−0.01	0.01	−0.02	7.41
Comment: changes in *net pH* are *normal*								
6.	7.02	61	15.8	12.5	−0.38	−0.08	−0.30	7.32
Comment: changes in *net pH (acidic)* are *mainly* due to *metabolic* component and *partly* due to *respiratory* component								

S. no	pH	pCO_2	HCO_3	Std HCO_3	pH-7.4	ΔRpH	ΔNRpH NRPH-7.4	Pr RpH 7.4 + ΔRpH
7.	7.5	57	44.5	39.3	0.1	−0.10	0.20	7.30
Comment: changes in *net pH (alkaline)* are *mainly* due to *metabolic* component, *partly opposed* by *respiratory* component (*acidic effect*)								
8.	7.4	72	44.6	36.1	0	−0.17	0.17	7.23
Comment: changes in *net pH* are *zero*. The changes in pH due to *metabolic* and *respiratory* component are *equal* and *opposite*. So, they *cancelled out each other* and the net change is zero								
9.	7.17	76	27.7	23.3	−0.23	−0.21	−0.02	7.19
Comment: changes in *net pH (acidic)* are *mainly* due to *respiratory* component								
10.	7.6	12	11.8	19.5	0.2	0.30	−0.10	7.70
Comment: changes in *net pH (alkaline)* are *mainly* due to *respiratory* component, *partly opposed* by *metabolic* component (*acidic effect*)								
11.	7.02	14	3.6	4.1	−0.38	0.40	−0.78	7.80
Comment: changes in *net pH (acidic)* are *mainly* due to *metabolic* component, *partly opposed* by *respiratory* component (*alkaline effect*)								

Table 1.
Examples of ABG data showing metabolic and respiratory components involved in net changes in total pH.

ABG interpretation because it is not routinely applied at the clinical practice due to the lack of simple formulae to calculate the same and nonavailability of its interrelationship with the other acid-base parameters. In the recently published research study, calculation of non-respiratory hydrogen ion concentration from standard bicarbonate and its relationship with other commonly utilized ABG parameters were discussed with the postulates of the acid-base balance theory and shown in **Figures 5–10** and *tabulated* in **Table 1** [14, 18].

5. Predicted respiratory pH

The predicted respiratory pH is usually calculated by pCO_2 variance. This calculation is slightly different for higher (>40 mmHg) and lower (<40 mmHg) pCO_2

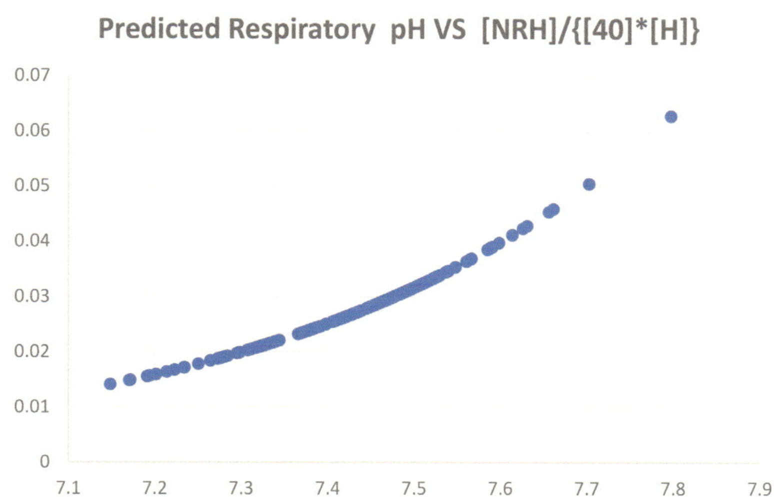

Figure 11.
X-axis predicted respiratory pH vs. y-axis [NRH]/{[40][H]}.*

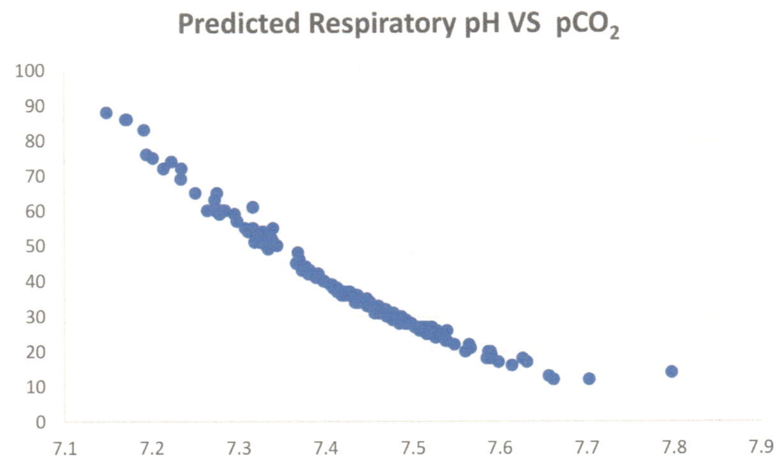

Figure 12.
X-axis predicted respiratory pH vs. y-axis pCO_2.

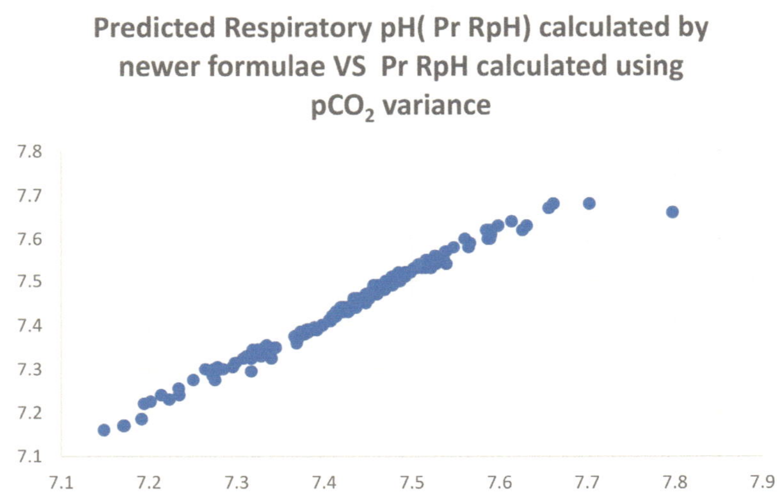

Figure 13.
X-axis predicted respiratory pH(Pr RpH) calculated by newer formulae vs. y-axis Pr RpH calculated using pCO_2 variance.

Predicted respiratory pH calculation using pCO_2 variance (previous method)		
Parameter	**$pCO_2 > 40$ mmHg**	**$pCO_2 < 40$ mmHg**
pCO_2 variance	$(pCO_2 - 40)/100$	$(40 - pCO_2)/100$
Predicted respiratory pH	$7.4 - (pCO_2 \text{ variance})/2$	$7.4 + (pCO_2 \text{ variance})$
Predicted respiratory pH calculation using newly derived formulae		
	Formulae is the same for all the values of PCO_2	
ΔRpH	$[pH - NRpH] = 1.6 + \log\{(HCO_3/\text{Std } HCO_3)/pCO_2\}$	
Predicted respiratory pH	7.4 + ΔRpH	

Table 2.
Comparison of predicted respiratory pH calculation (one by previous method using pCO_2 variance and the other by newly derived formulae).

levels. The difference between the predicted respiratory pH and the measured pH reflects the metabolic pH change. [15] The predicted respiratory pH is calculated by using a newly derived formula which is common for all pCO_2 values [18]. The graphical relationship is shown in **Figures 11–13** and tabulated in **Table 2**.

6. Postulates of the acid-base balance theory

The postulates of the acid-base balance theory are listed below [14]:

1. The net changes in pH of the blood reflect the sum total changes in the hydrogen ion concentration in the blood. The net changes in total or actual pH [ΔpH (pH − 7.4)] are due to both the changes in respiratory [ΔRpH (pH − NRpH)] and non-respiratory (metabolic) components [ΔNRpH (NRpH − 7.4)] affecting the pH.

2. The sum total changes in the hydrogen ion concentration ($\Delta H + = [H^+] - [40]$) in the blood include both the changes due to respiratory ($\Delta RH^+ = [H^+] - [NRH^+]$) and non-respiratory (metabolic) components ($\Delta NRH^+ = [NRH^+] - [40]$).

3. The non-respiratory hydrogen ion concentration [NRH^+] has a unique value for a given standard bicarbonate concentration represented by the relation $NRH^+ = 960/\text{Std bicarbonate}$.

4. The concentration of hydrogen ion excess given by [$NRH^+ - 40$] is directly proportional to the base deficit. This quantity with opposite sign [$40 - NRH^+$] is directly proportional to the base excess. Standard base excess is the base excess at hemoglobin concentration of 5 g/dl.

5. The changes in the dependent variable non-respiratory hydrogen ion concentration [NRH^+] representing the non-respiratory (metabolic) component are due to the changes by the independent variables, namely, strong ion difference (SID) and the total concentration of weak nonvolatile acids, namely, albumin and phosphate [ATOT].

6. The changes in the dependent variable [HCO_3] are a marker of metabolic acid-base disturbances and not its causative mechanism.

7. The magnitude and direction (positive or negative) of the changes in the parameter ΔNRpH(NRpH − 7.4) are due to the accumulation of acids other than carbonic acid or bases. The value is negative for acidic effect and positive for alkaline effect.

8. The magnitude and direction (positive or negative) of the changes in the parameter ΔRpH(pH − NRpH) denote the respiratory influence in causing changes in pH represented by the relation $pH - NRpH = 1.6 + \log\{(HCO_3/\text{Std } HCO_3)/pCO_2\}$. The value is negative for acidic effect and positive for alkaline effect.

9. The ratio [NRH^+/H^+] is directly proportional to the parameter ΔRpH (pH − NRpH) which denotes the respiratory influence of pCO_2.

10. The respiratory influence of pCO_2 in changing pH through bicarbonate is a variable one (ratio of HCO_3/Std HCO_3) depending on the acute or chronic conditions or compensations and through carbonic acid is a constant one given by $(H_2CO_3 - 1.2)/H_2CO_3$.

7. Conclusion

Arterial blood gas analysis test is one of the most commonly employed point-of-care testings in intensive care units, yet the understanding of acid-base disturbances and interpretation of ABG reports are sometimes a challenging task especially for critically ill patients with multiorgan failure. The graphical relationship between the metabolic and respiratory components of the net changes in pH and the total changes in hydrogen ion concentration with other ABG parameters like standard base excess, bicarbonate, standard bicarbonate, and pCO_2 will help in better understanding of the arterial blood gas interpretation which results in proper, quicker, and better management of the patient's critical conditions. A newer graphical tool developed using standard base excess and the ratio of (HCO_3 – standard HCO_3)/ H_2CO_3 may help in easier and quicker interpretation of ABG reports. This simple four-quadrant graph method may provide a rough guide for ABG interpretation, which, when applied at the appropriate time, results in timely management.

Although, standard bicarbonate value is not routinely utilized for ABG interpretation, the parameters derived from standard bicarbonate plays a vital role in the understanding of acid-base disturbances. The application of these newly derived parameters and the four-quadrant graphical tool may serve as a supporting tool for teaching and diagnostic purposes, which when properly correlated with clinical conditions and other ABG parameters results in better understanding and quicker interpretation of ABG reports.

Conflict of interest

Nil.

Author details

T. Rajini Samuel
Shri Sathya Sai Medical College and Research Institute, Sri Balaji Vidyapeeth Deemed to be University, Kancheepuram District, Tamilnadu, India

*Address all correspondence to: samuel.biochemistry@gmail.com; samuel.rajini@ gmail.com

References

[1] Samuel RA. Graphical tool for arterial blood gas interpretation using standard bicarbonate and base excess. Indian journal of Medical Biochemistry. 2018; **22**(1):85-89

[2] Samuel R, Ilanchezian, Rajagopalan B. Application of modified Henderson equation in ABG interpretation. International Journal of Pharmaceutical Sciences Review and Research. 2016; **37**(2):169-177

[3] Arterial Blood Gases—Indications and Interpretation. 2010. Available from: Patient.info/doctor [Accessed: February, 10 2013]

[4] Baillie K. Arterial Blood Gas Interpreter. Online: Arterial Blood Gas Analysis. Available from: prognosis.org [Accessed: July 05, 2007]

[5] Marino PL. Arterial Blood Gas Interpretation. 2nd edi ed. Philadelphia: Lippincott/Williams and Wilkins Publishers; 1998. pp. 582-605

[6] Narins RG, Emmett M. Simple and mixed acid-base disorders: A practical approach. Medicine. 1980;**59**:161-187

[7] Adrogue HJ. Mixed acid-base disturbances. Journal of Nephrology. 2006;**19**(Suppl 9):S97-S103

[8] Siggaard-Andersen O, Fogh-Andersen N. Base excess or buffer base (strong ion difference) as measure of a non-respiratory acid-base disturbance. Acta Anaesthesiologica Scandinavica. 1995;**39**(Supplementum 106):123-128

[9] Mizock BA. Utility of standard base excess in acid-base analysis. Critical Care Medicine. 1998;**26**(7):1146-1147

[10] Siggaard-Andersen O. Acid-base balance. In: Boston GEO, editor. Encyclopedia of Respiratory Medicine. Amsterdam: Academic Press; 2006. pp. 5-10

[11] Jørgensen K, Astrup P. Standard bicarbonate, its clinical significance, and a new method for its determination. Scandinavian Journal of Clinical & Laboratory Investigation. 1957;**9**(2): 122-132

[12] Krapf R. Standard bicarbonate and base excess-obsolete parameter. Therapeutische Umschau. 2000;**57**(6): 386-390

[13] Suero JT. The usefulness of non-respiratory hydrogen ion concentration and its relationship to the traditional acid-base parameters. Clinical Biochemistry. 1969;**2**:177-185

[14] Rajini Samuel T. Application and inter-relationship of non-respiratory hydrogen ion concentration in acid-base balance theory. International Journal of Clinical Chemistry and Laboratory Medicine (IJCCLM). 2018;**4**(3):1-13

[15] Munjal YP, Surendra K, Sharm API. Section 7: Critical care medicine. Chapter 4: Acid base disorders. In: Textbook of Medicine. Ninth ed. 2012. pp. 239-241

[16] Whitehead TP. Acid-base status, pH, and PCO_2. Lancet. 1965;**2**:1015-1016

[17] Bookallil MJ. Description of pH or Acid-Base Status in Blood, pH of the Blood: Acid Base Balance. Available from: www.anaesthesia.med.usyd.edu.au/resources/lectures/acidbase_mjb/acidbase.html

[18] Samuel R. A graphical representation for aiding arterial blood gas interpretation using non-respiratory and respiratory pH. World Journal of Pharmaceutical and Medical Research. 2018;**4**(12):192-202

Chapter 5

Red Blood Cells as Redox Modulators in Hemolytic Anemia

Eitan Fibach and Mutaz Dana

Abstract

The oxidative status of cells, representing the balance between prooxidants and antioxidants, is involved in their normal physiological functioning, such as signal transduction, proliferation, and differentiation. When the prooxidant activity overrides the antioxidative capacity oxidative stress occurs. Chronic oxidative stress causes cytotoxicity and organ failure. As such, it is believed to play a role in various pathologies, including the hemolytic anemias. In this review, we suggest that red blood cells (RBC), in addition to their primary role as oxygen carriers, function as redox modulators. In the RBC, various systems afford it with antioxidative capacity that, in addition to balancing its own redox state, can provide antioxidative protection to the cellular and intracellular milieus throughout the body. Their vast number, mobility, occurrence throughout the body, and renewability make them good candidates for this function. A decrease in their number (anemia) or function due to oxidative stress may exacerbate the symptoms of many diseases by failing to neutralize oxidative stress. However, correcting anemia, e.g., by repeated RBC transfusions or iron supplementation, may increase the iron load, which, in turn, causes oxidative stress. This situation suggests that the status of both iron and redox should be monitored during treatment, using RBC as bioindicators.

Keywords: red blood cells, hemolytic anemia, thalassemia, oxidative stress, flow cytometry

1. Introduction

The redox status of cells is crucial for normal physiological functioning; however, when the prooxidant activity overrides the antioxidative capacity (AOC), oxidative stress occurs. Chronic oxidative stress causes cytotoxicity and organ failure. As such, it is believed to play a role in many diseases, such as cardiovascular, thromboembolic and neurodegenerative disorders, as well as aging [1].

In this review, we suggest that RBC, in addition to their primary role as oxygen and CO_2 carriers, functions as redox modulators. Various RBC systems afford them with AOC that, in addition to balancing their own redox state, can provide antioxidative protection to the cellular and intercellular milieus throughout the body. Their vast number, mobility, and occurrence throughout the body and renewability make them good candidates for this function. A decrease in their number (anemia) or function may exacerbate the symptoms of many diseases by failing to neutralize oxidative stress. However, correcting anemia, e.g., by repeated RBC transfusions or by iron supplementation, may increase the iron load, which, in turn, causes oxidative stress. This situation suggests that the status of both iron and redox should be monitored during treatment, using RBC as bioindicators.

2. Oxidative stress and its involvement in pathology

The cellular redox status represents the balance between generation of free radicals, such as the reactive oxygen species (ROS) and reactive nitrogen species (RNS), and the ability to detoxify them or to repair their resultant damage by antioxidants, such as the reduced glutathione (GSH), the major intracellular scavenger of ROS. ROS are generated in cells mainly during energy production: In the mitochondria, about 2% of the total oxygen (O_2) consumption results in the free radical superoxide anion (O_2^-) [1]. While not particularly reactive, superoxide can act as a reductant toward divalent metal ions, mainly iron and copper, and can react with itself by spontaneous or enzymatic (e.g., by the reducing enzyme superoxide dismutase, SOD) dismutation to form hydrogen peroxide (H_2O_2). The latter is a mild oxidant, but in the presence of divalent metals, it can generate the reactive hydroxyl ($^{\cdot}OH$) radical.

In mature RBC, which are devoid of mitochondria, the hemoglobin (Hb) is the major source of ROS generation [2]. The heme iron, which is in the Fe(II) ferrous state in the oxygenated Hb, is oxidized to the Fe(III) ferric state in metHb—a reaction that normally occurs at a rate of about 3% of the Hb per day. This process results in the production of superoxide that in turn generates hydrogen peroxide and oxygen as products of dismutation by SOD [3]. The metHb is then restored back to oxyHb by the NADH-cytochrome b5 reductase [4].

An additional pathway of oxygen to superoxide reduction is by nicotinamide adenine dinucleotide phosphate (NADPH) oxidases. Phagocytic cells, such as polymorphonuclear (PMN) neutrophils and macrophages, have an NADPH oxidase complex that generates ROS as part of the innate immune response to infection. Non-phagocytic cells contain NADPH oxidases that generate ROS, at lower levels than phagocytes, for signaling responses [5]. ROS can also arise as the indirect by-product of enzymatic activities, such as that of monooxygenases (e.g., cytochrome P450) [6].

RNS originate from the gaseous molecule nitric oxide (NO). The latter is synthesized by constitutive or inducible nitric oxide synthase enzymes by oxidation of L-arginine to L-citrulline. NO can react rapidly with the superoxide anion to form the oxidant peroxynitrite ($ONOO^-$), nitrogen dioxide (NO_2), nitroxyl (HNO), and nitrosonium cation (NO^+) (for review see [7]).

The cellular prooxidants are tightly controlled by restricting the magnitude and the location of their generation and by elaborating antioxidant mechanisms that scavenge their excess and correct their toxic consequences (for review see [1]). In addition to these intracellular antioxidant mechanisms, extracellular mechanisms function as well. For example, the blood serum contains many molecules with AOC such as bilirubin, albumin, ascorbic acid, as well as diet-derived antioxidants such as polyphenols.

Under certain conditions, excess oxidants my override the AOC and generate a state of oxidative stress. This may occur due to external factors (e.g., certain food components, air pollution, sun exposure, environmental radiation, as well as radio- and chemotherapeutic regimes) or internal factors such as various pathological circumstances (e.g., inflammation, iron overload, Hb instability). Excess ROS react quickly with bio-molecules such as the DNA, proteins, and lipids, interfering with cellular functions. As such, even if it is not the primary etiology, oxidative stress is believed to mediate the symptoms of many diseases, such as cancer, atherosclerosis, diabetes, cardiovascular, thromboembolic and neurodegenerative disorders, as well as physiological aging [1].

3. Hemolytic anemia

We have studied oxidative stress in hemolytic anemias [8]. The anemia in these hereditary or acquired diseases is the result of augmented destruction (hemolysis) of mature RBC and their immature progenitors/precursors that is not balanced by compensatory overproduction. Among these diseases are: (I) The hemoglobinopathies—caused by mutations in the globin genes, leading to insufficient production (thalassemia) or production of aborted (sickle cell disease) globin chains [9]. (II) RBC membrane/cytoskeletal disorders such as hereditary spherocytosis, elliptocytosis, and stomatocytosis—caused by mutations in genes leading to abnormal RBC shape and propensity for hemolysis [10]. (III) Inherited enzymatic defects in RBC such as glucose-6-phosphate dehydrogenase (G6PD) deficiency and pyruvate kinase deficiency. G6PD is a key enzyme of the pentose pathway (hexose monophosphate shunt) which supplies NADPH—a reducing agent that is important for the regulation of the redox state, especially in RBC [11]. Patients with G6PD deficiency exhibit hemolytic anemia in response to infection and certain medications or foods. (IV) Paroxysmal nocturnal hemoglobinuria—a clonal disease caused by an acquired somatic mutation in the phosphatidylinositol glycan complementation class A gene. This gene encodes the enzyme responsible for the first step in the production of the glycosylphosphatidylinositol anchor, by which various proteins are linked to the plasma membrane. In this disease, the mutation occurs in a hematopoietic stem cell and is expressed in its progeny, affecting various membrane proteins including the complement (C′) inhibitors: CD55 (decay-accelerating factor) which inhibits the C3 component of the C′, and CD59 (membrane inhibitor of reactive lysis) which inhibits terminal C′ components (C5b-9) from forming the hemolytic membrane pore [12]. This leads to hemolysis and platelet activation, leading to anemia and to venous thrombosis, respectively [13]. (V) Congenital dyserythropoietic anemias—a heterogeneous group of diseases characterized by anemia due to abnormalities of erythroid precursor cells and reduced erythropoiesis [14]. (VI) Autoimmune hemolytic anemia such as ABO mismatch transfusion reaction and severe idiopathic autoimmune hemolytic anemia—caused by autoantibodies against antigens expressed on the surface of RBC. Once formed, these antibodies bind to the surface of RBC marking them for destruction through C′-mediated lysis (intravascular hemolysis) and/or Fc-mediated phagocytosis (extravascular hemolysis). Autoimmune hemolytic anemia can occur alone, but is often seen in association with other autoimmune diseases, cancer, drug treatment, transfusion, and pregnancy. (VII) Myelodysplastic syndromes (MDS)—diverse conditions that involve ineffective production (dysplasia) of hematopoietic cells. The patients often develop severe anemia and require frequent blood transfusions. In most cases, the disease worsens, and the patient develops cytopenias due to progressive bone marrow failure. In about one third of patients, the disease transforms into acute myelogenous leukemia, usually within months to a few years.

Although oxidative stress is not the primary etiology of these diseases, except for G6PD deficiency, it mediates their symptoms, including anemia, recurrent infections, and thromboembolic complications [8]. The main causes of oxidative stress in these diseases are: (I) Degradation of abnormal Hbs in the mature RBC and their precursors (in the hemoglobinopathies), leading to the production of hemichromes and eventually to release of heme and iron. (II) Iron overload caused by frequent blood transfusions and increased iron uptake [15]. Usually, iron uptake in the gut as well as its mobilization from storage cells, regulated by hepcidin, is downregulated by iron excess [16]. It these diseases, where the body attempts to compensate for the anemia by over production of new RBC ("ineffective erythropoiesis"), iron is in high demand. To ensure sufficient iron uptake, the developing erythroid progenitors produce factors that inhibit hepcidin production, thus overriding the regulating effect of hepcidin. (III) Iron-containing compounds (Hb and hemin) which are released by intravascular hemolysis can also add to the iron load and further aggravate the hemolysis [17]. In the absence of specific mechanisms for disposal of excess iron, under these conditions iron accumulates. Iron overload increases ROS generation by catalyzing the Haber-Weiss/Fenton biochemical reactions [3, 18].

4. RBC as redox modulators

The main function of RBC is oxygen transport, for which they have evolved efficient nonenzymatic and enzymatic antioxidative systems for protection against oxidizing substances to which they are exposed. The nonenzymatic systems include reduced glutathione, thioredoxin, ascorbic acid, and vitamin E. The most important antioxidant enzymes include SOD, thioredoxin reductase/peroxiredoxin system, catalase, glutathione peroxidase, glutathione reductase, plasma membrane oxidoreductases, and the metHb reductase/NADH/glycolysis system that maintains Hb in a Fe(II)-active form [19].

Although these systems mainly serve the RBC own requirements, it seems that since they are produced in excess they can be utilized for antioxidant protection of other cells, at least under conditions of oxidative stress. This function may affect the intra- and extracellular milieus throughout the body, especially of cells in the circulation and in the perivascular tissues (endothelial cells).

Several characteristics, in addition to their extra reducing power, make RBC ideal candidates to serve as redox mediators. These include their vast number, mobility, and occurrence throughout the body. The consequence of their antioxidative activity could be oxidative damage to the RBC themself, facilitating their erythrophagocytosis, degradation, and detoxification of their oxidized constituents by macrophages in reticuloendothelial systems, mainly the spleen and the liver. These damaged/old RBC are replaced by new RBC that are continuously formed in the bone marrow.

A "bystander" effect of cells on the oxidative status of other neighboring cells has been described previously in other circumstances of oxidative stress induced by ionizing or photoradiation [20, 21].

4.1 Proofs of the concept

The concept of the RBC protective role was first introduced by Fazi et al. [22]. They showed that RBC are able to inactivate harmful xenobiotics, including 1-chloro-2,4-dinitrobenzene, by conjugation with glutathione and suggested that it may be possible to treat xenobiotic intoxication by transfusion of GSH-loaded RBC.

Richards et al. have shown that RBC can protect endothelial cells from PMN-induced damage [23]. PMN exert their antibacterial effect by generating a burst of ROS (respiratory burst) in response to toxins released by phagocytosed bacteria. These ROS not only kill the bacteria but also damage the PMN themselves and other neighboring cells (inflammation). The respiratory burst can be reproduced in vitro by incubating PMN with phorbol myristate acetate (PMA). In their study, ^{51}Cr-labeled endothelial cells were incubated with PMA-triggered PMN. Damage to the endothelial cells was measured by the release of ^{51}Cr into the incubation medium. Adding RBC to the mixture reduced the damage dose-dependently. Analyzing the RBC following the incubation, revealed reduced levels of 2,3-diphosphoglyceric acid and glutathione, and increased levels of the oxidation products malondialdehyde and metHb. These results indicated that these RBC are under oxidative stress compared with RBC incubated alone or with non-triggered PMN. The authors suggested that RBC can provide antioxidant protection to other tissues in vivo [24].

We have studied the effect of RBC on the oxidative status of other cells by measuring oxidative parameters by flow cytometry. Following pulse-labeling of cells with the probe 2′7′-dichlorodihydrofluorescindiacetate, their fluorescence was proportional to their ROS content. The increase in their fluorescence after washing indicated their rate of generation of ROS. In our experiments, the labeled cells were incubated with RBC derived from either normal donors or patients with β-thalassemia. Normal RBC had a dose-dependent decrease effect on ROS generation, while thalassemic RBC had a much inferior effect [25].

It is well known that thalassemic RBC are under oxidative stress and contain more free iron load (the labile iron pool) than normal RBC [26]. To explore this condition on their AOC, RBC were exposed to agents that affect their oxidative stress or iron overload: normal RBC—to the oxidant hydrogen peroxide or to an iron source, ferric ammonium citrate, and thalassemic RBC—to the antioxidant N-acetyl cysteine or to the iron chelator, Desferal. The RBC were then mixed with the probe-labeled cells, and the kinetics of ROS generated by the labeled cells was monitored during incubation. The results indicated that oxidants and iron reduced the AOC of RBC (**Figure 1**).

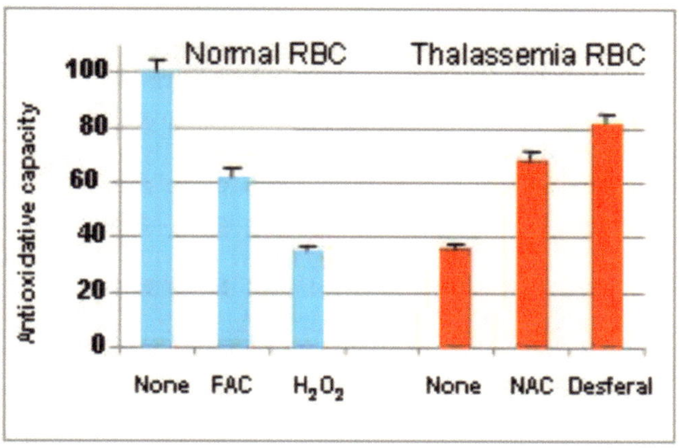

Figure 1.
The effects of iron overload and oxidative stress on the antioxidative capacity (AOC) of normal and thalassemia RBC. The human myeloid leukemia HL60 cells were labeled with 2′-7′-di-chlorofluorescein diacetate, washed, and then incubated with 6×10^6/ml RBC from normal or β-thalassemia donors (N = 6 each). Prior to incubation with cells, the RBC had been treated for 30 min: normal RBC with ferric ammonium citrate (FAC), 1 mM, and thalassemic RBC—with the iron chelator, Desferal, 5 mM—thus increasing and decreasing iron overload, respectively. Alternatively, normal RBC had been treated with the oxidant H_2O_2, 5 mM, and thalassemic RBCs—with the anti-oxidant N-acetyl cysteine (NAC), 5 mM—thus increasing and decreasing oxidative stress, respectively. The cells were then analyzed by a flow cytometer (FACS-calibur^R; Becton-Dickinson, Immunofluorometry systems, Mountain View, CA, USA). The average (mean fluorescence channel) cellular green fluorescence (FL-1), reversely indicating the AOC, of 40,000 HL60 cells, was determined. In the analysis, RBC were excluded from HL60 cells by gating based on forward - and side-light scatter and fluorescence. The results indicate that the AOC of thalassemia RBC was significantly lower than that of normal RBC, and that iron and oxidants further decreased it, but it could be restored by iron chelation or antioxidants.

4.2 RBC as oxidants

Oxidative stress, being a common feature of many diseases, affects most cells of the body, including the RBC. These diseases involve RBC directly (e.g., thalassemia) or indirectly (e.g., diabetes) [27]. We have shown oxidative stress in RBC in all the hemolytic anemias [15]. Oxidative stress in RBC diminishing their own AOC, resulting in their short survival, but also reduces their ability to protect other cells. Under extreme conditions, this situation may turn the RBC into oxidative agents, rather than antioxidative agents.

4.3 Probable mechanisms involved in redox protection of RBC

Using artificial vesicles, it has been shown that while hydrogen peroxide readily crosses biological membranes, superoxide does it very slowly [28]. Vesicles made of RBC membranes allow superoxide to cross through and oxidize cytochrome c in the suspending medium within a time-frame consistent with its half-life time [29]. This transfer probably occurs via an anion channel since it was inhibited by stilbenes, which inhibit the exchange of anions across the membrane. Whether such outward flux actually occurs in intact RBC is doubtful. Since RBC contain a large amount of SOD [30], it seems unlikely that superoxide made within the RBC would escape both the spontaneous and enzymatic dismutations and diffuse across the membrane. In contrast, an inward flux could occur. The plasma contains comparatively little SOD [31], and superoxides generated outside the RBC might diffuse inward to be scavenged by the RBC-SOD. In this fashion, RBC might limit the damage inflicted by superoxides produced by blood phagocytes and vascular endothelial cells.

Similarly, RBC provide a mechanism for inactivation of free NO [32]. NO liberated from endothelium may be taken up by RBC and inactivated by oxyHb that in turn is converted to metHb, while the NO is converted to nitrate to be secreted by the kidneys.

Another RBC redox protective mechanism involves ascorbic acid (AA) (vitamin C) [33]. In humans, AA dietary intake is essential for maintaining plasma and tissue reductive capacity. It primarily functions to scavenge superoxide anion and singlet oxygen, but it also removes other ROS generated by protein-bound redox metals and xanthine oxidase. AA itself is oxidized to an AA radical and dehydro AA. Human RBC were suggested to possess a two-layered system of redox recycling of low concentrations of the AA radical under minimal oxidative stress and a backup system of recycling of large quantities of dehydro AA under increased oxidative stress. RBC accumulation of dehydro AA as a result of prooxidative conditions originates in part outside of the RBC during the two-electron oxidation of AA, which is subsequently transported reversibly in competition with glucose by the type 1 glucose transporters spanning the RBC membrane. Alternatively, dehydro AA may be lost altogether by degradation, removing a pool of potentially reversible oxidized AA. Experimental evidence suggests that recycling of AA by the RBC significantly add to the AOC of the blood [34].

Still another potential RBC redox protective mechanism is through the release of antioxidants and antioxidative enzymes (e.g., SOD and catalase) following hemolysis. We have found that hemolysate inhibits ROS generation by cells (unpublished observation). This could also occur following shedding of membrane-bound vesicles during the maturation of erythroid precursors in the bone marrow and senescence of RBC in the circulation. Both processes are enhanced in hemolytic anemias by oxidative stress [35].

Except for direct effects, RBC may affect other cells indirectly. For example, diet-derived antioxidant polyamines tend to attach to RBC membranes, resulting in a synergistic enhancement of their antioxidative activity [36].

5. Pathological significance of RBC as redox modulators

The redox-modulating activity of RBC could affect cells and their function throughout the body. We have studied their effect on platelets. Hemolytic anemia, such as thalassemia, is often associated with high incidence of thromboembolic complications (e.g., venous thrombosis and stroke) due to platelet hyperactivation and plasma hypercoagulation [37]. Platelet functioning depends on their redox state. They have an inherent ability to produce ROS by various pathways—as a by-product of the mitochondrial respiratory chain [38] and by the NADH/NADPH oxidase [for a review see [39]] produced mainly in the pentose cycle [40]. ROS, along with NO, adenosine, and prostacyclins, may play a profound role in the regulation of platelet activities [41]. Many studies demonstrated that their functioning during clot formation involves ROS; for example, platelet activators, such as thrombin, increase ROS generation [42–44].

Oxidative stress in platelets may give rise to two pathological outcomes: (I) toxicity, resulting in thrombocytopenia and bleeding and (II) hyperactivation resulting in excess clot formation leading to thromboembolic complications. Exemplifying the latter is hydrogen peroxide that stimulates their oxidative stress [45], and affects their various functions: activation by: (I) arachidonic acid and collagen [46]; (II) thrombin and ADP [47–49]; (III) tyrosine phosphorylation of the platelet $\alpha IIb\beta 3$, an independent platelet activation pathway, thereby enhancing their aggregation [50], as well as (IV) through scavenging of the platelet- or endothelium-derived NO—thereby decreasing its aggregation-inhibiting effect [51]. Superoxide can also contribute to late clot growth by increasing the bioavailability of ADP and subsequently recruiting additional platelets [49].

Since platelets do not carry known specific inherent redox pathology, it is reasonable to attribute their oxidative stress, at least in part, to continuous exposure to oxidative insults from extra platelet sources, such as their environment, i.e., the blood plasma, and neighboring cells - blood cells and the vascular endothelium. We have shown that incubation of normal platelets with plasma from thalassemia patients, rather than with normal plasma, resulted in their oxidative stress and activation [52]. Potential plasma oxidants are iron-containing compounds such as non-transferrin-bound iron, ferritin, heme, or Hb, all of which are increased in thalassemia patients [47, 53]. Incubation of platelets with iron (ferric ammonium citrate), heme (hemin or heme arginate), or Hb stimulated their oxidative stress. Moreover, addition of the iron-chelator deferoxamine to thalassemic plasma reduced its effect on the platelets' ROS [52].

Interestingly, thalassemic RBC also increased normal platelet oxidative status. In contrast, normal RBC, unless treated with oxidants, decreased it [54]. These results suggest that thalassemic RBC, having a higher than normal ROS level, mediate oxidative stress in platelets directly, probably by contact or close proximity [25]. These results are compatible with studies showing that platelets could be activated by ROS generated by neighboring cells such as RBC, neutrophils [55, 56], fibroblasts, and vascular endothelial and smooth muscle cells [39].

RBC might also affect platelets indirectly by a variety of mechanisms: (I) Release of iron-containing oxidants into the plasma [46, 57, 58], as mentioned above. (II) Release of ROS, e.g., superoxide anions, causing oxidation of low-density lipoprotein [59], which, in turn, might activate platelets [60]. (III) Exposure or shedding of phosphatidylserine moieties, which act as a procoagulant that amplifies the generation of thrombin and thus initiates platelet activation [61]. Thalassemic RBC have been shown to carry and shed higher than normal levels of external phosphatidylserine [35].

Other important function of the RBC-AOC is to scavenge and detoxify NO, an important vasodilating agent. released from the vascular endothelial cells [32] and by inflamed tissues [62].

The role of RBC as redox modulators can be compromised under pathological conditions: when their number decrease (anemia) and when their AOC is defective, both of which may co-exist in many diseases. Anemia may elevate oxidative stress by reducing the oxygen availability (hypoxia) to tissue cells and by reducing the AOC of the RBC.

Various therapeutic modalities may be used to correct anemia:

- Iron supplementation in the case of deficiency.

- Administration of erythropoiesis-stimulating agents such as erythropoietin (EPO) in cases of reduced erythropoiesis. This includes patients with chronic kidney disease where there is insufficient EPO production due to renal dysfunction, patients with malignancies during the course of chemotherapy, and patients with myelodysplastic syndrome. In most of these cases, the treatment comprises both EPO and iron supplementation.

- Blood transfusion is used in the event of acute, severe, hemorrhage, or in chronic hemolysis. An example of the latter is β-thalassemia major where patients are transfused with packed RBC every 3 weeks for their entire life.

Both transfusions and EPO have been used pre- and post-major operative procedures that are associated with severe blood loss.

All these therapeutic procedures, on one hand, increase the RBC mass and thereby, supposedly, its AOC. On the other hand, iron supplementation and transfusions might increase the iron load leading to oxidative stress in cells, including RBC, thus compromising their AOC. For example, multi-transfused thalassemic patients, with less severe anemia but higher iron overload, have lower levels of oxidative stress (ROS and lipid hydroperoxides) than un-transfused patients, with more severe anemia but lower iron overload [63]. In cardiovascular diseases, although there is ample clinical evidence for the worsening effect of anemia, RBC transfusions or EPO administration were not always effective [64–66]. As for EPO, it has been demonstrated to have an antioxidative effect on various cells, including RBC [67], and thereby might increase their AOC. The net effect of anemia and iron overload on

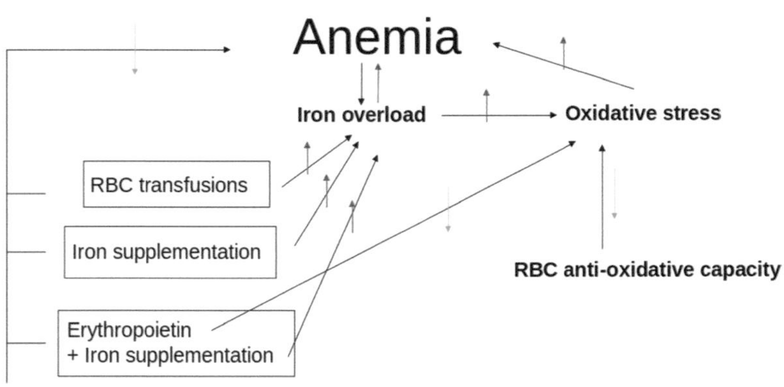

Figure 2.
The relationship among anemia, its treatment and RBC antioxidative capacity on oxidative stress. Upward red arrows indicate an increase; the downward blue arrows indicate a decrease.

oxidative stress warrants a careful study in transfused and non-transfused patients and favors continuous monitoring of the status of iron and oxidative stress during these treatments. This complex relationship is graphically summarized in **Figure 2**.

Some therapeutic protocols are used to reduce the RBC mass (hematocrit). Bloodletting (phlebotomy) is used in cases of polycythemia (erythrocytosis), either primary (polycythemia vera), familiar, or secondary [68], as well as hereditary hemochromatosis—an inheritable disease characterized by iron overload [69]. The benefit of this treatment with respect to decreasing the iron load should be weighed against its potential reducing effect of the RBC-AOC.

6. RBC as redox bioindicators

The oxidative state of RBC depends on intra-RBC factors such as enzymopahtology (e.g., G6PD deficiency), Hb instability (thalassemia and sickle cell disease), membrane pathology (hereditary spherocytosis), glucose metabolism [diabetes [27]], or extra-RBC factors such as in inflammation. Their oxidative state, in turn, may affect their AOC. It was suggested that RBC could be used as bioindicators of prognostic value in clinical practice [19]. They may provide a real-time monitoring of their own conditions as well as those in other parts of the body. This is potentially relevant to RBC-linked and unlinked pathologic conditions associated with oxidative stress.

6.1 Measurement of the redox status in RBC

Measurement of redox parameters in cells and in body fluids, such as the blood plasma, can be accomplished by various methods [3]. These measurements, however, are not a common practice in the clinic mainly because the methodologies are inadequate for the routine clinical laboratory. We have measured redox parameters [54, 70], including the labile iron pool [71], in RBC by flow cytometry, a common methodology in the clinical setting. Various fluorescent probes have been used. For example, ROS were measured by 2′7′-dichlorodihydrofluorescindiacetate, [72]. Following free diffusion into cells, this nonfluorescent compound is esterified and gets trapped intracellularly as 2′7′-dichlorodihydrofluorescein. ROS, mainly peroxides, oxidize it to the fluorescent derivative 2′7′-dichlorodihydrofluorescein that its cellular fluorescence is proportional to ROS generation [72].

Several points should be considered using this method: (I) Since ROS are short-lived, analyses should be performed on fresh samples. (II) The probes used are not specific to a particular ROS—a limitation that does not limit the assessment of general oxidative stress. (III) The intracellular probe content depends on the experimental settings: the concentration of probe added to the composition of the medium and the incubation conditions, such as the temperature. However, it also depends on the cellular uptake of the probe and its esterification, which depends on the different properties of cells (e.g., activated vs. inactivated, pathological vs. normal). To overcome these caveats, we have modified the protocol: Cells were pulsed with the probe, washed, and then re-incubated in probe-free medium. The kinetics of ROS generation was determined by measuring the cellular fluorescence at different times.

The method was validated by determining the effect on RBC fluorescence of the ROS-generating agent peroxide, the catalase inhibitor sodium azide, and the ROS scavenger N-acetyl cysteine. When normal RBC were compared with RBC from β-thalassemia patients, both the basal fluorescence and its kinetics were higher in the latter, confirming that thalassemic RBC were under oxidative stress.

7. Conclusions

The redox state is crucial for physiological functioning of cells, but excess reactive oxygen and nitrogen species causes oxidative stress, which is associated with many diseases, including hemolytic anemia. These anemias are characterized by accelerated destruction (hemolysis) of mature RBC and their precursors that is not balanced by compensatory overproduction. Although oxidative stress is not the primary etiology of most of these anemias, it mediates many of their symptoms. The main function of RBC is oxygen transport, for which they have evolved efficient nonenzymatic and enzymatic antioxidative systems for protection against oxidizing substances to which they are exposed. These systems serve mainly the RBC requirements, but may influence other neighboring cells as well, making the RBC antioxidative protective agents of the cellular and intracellular milieus throughout the body. Their vast number, mobility, occurrence throughout the body and renewability make them good candidates for this function. A decrease in their number (anemia) or function may exacerbate the symptoms of many diseases, including hemolytic anemias, by failing to neutralize oxidative stress. However, correcting anemia, e.g., by repeated RBC transfusions or iron supplementation, may increase the iron load, which, in turn, causes oxidative stress. This situation suggests that the status of both iron and redox should be monitored during treatment, using RBC as bioindicators and using flow cytometry multiparameter analysis.

Conflict of interest

The authors have no conflict of interests.

Author details

Eitan Fibach* and Mutaz Dana
Department of Hematology, Hadassah–Hebrew University Medical Center, Jerusalem, Israel

*Address all correspondence to: fibach@yahoo.com

References

[1] Halliwell B, Gutteridge J. Free Radicals in Biology and Medicine. 3rd ed. Midsomer Norton, Avon, England: Oxford University Press; 1999

[2] Rifkind JM, Nagababu E, Ramasamy S, Ravi LB. Hemoglobin redox reactions and oxidative stress. Redox Report. 2003;**8**(5):234-237

[3] Kohen R, Nyska A. Oxidation of biological systems: Oxidative stress phenomena, antioxidants, redox reactions, and methods for their quantification. Toxicologic Pathology. 2002;**30**(6):620-650

[4] Elahian F, Sepehrizadeh Z, Moghimi B, Mirzaei SA. Human cytochrome b5 reductase: Structure, function, and potential applications. Critical Reviews in Biotechnology. 2014;**34**(2):134-143

[5] Martindale JL, Holbrook NJ. Cellular response to oxidative stress: Signaling for suicide and survival. Journal of Cellular Physiology. 2002;**192**(1):1-15

[6] Wolke C, Bukowska A, Goette A, Lendeckel U. Redox control of cardiac remodeling in atrial fibrillation. Biochimica et Biophysica Acta. 2015;**1850**(8):1555-1565

[7] Martinez MC, Andriantsitohaina R. Reactive nitrogen species: Molecular mechanisms and potential significance in health and disease. Antioxidants & Redox Signaling. 2009;**11**(3):669-702

[8] Fibach E, Rachmilewitz E. The role of oxidative stress in hemolytic anemia. Current Molecular Medicine. 2008;**8**(7):609-619

[9] Weatherall DJ. Phenotype-genotype relationships in monogenic disease: Lessons from the thalassaemias. Nature Reviews. Genetics. 2001;**2**(4):245-255

[10] Da Costa L, Galimand J, Fenneteau O, Mohandas N. Hereditary spherocytosis, elliptocytosis, and other red cell membrane disorders. Blood Reviews. 2013;**27**(4):167-178

[11] Luzzatto L, Battistuzzi G. Glucose-6-phosphate dehydrogenase. Advances in Human Genetics. 1985;**14**:217, 86-329, 88

[12] Walport MJ. Complement. First of two parts. The New England Journal of Medicine. 2001;**344**(14):1058-1066

[13] Parker CJ. The pathophysiology of paroxysmal nocturnal hemoglobinuria. Experimental Hematology. 2007;**35**(4):523-533

[14] Shalev H, Al-Athamen K, Levi I, Levitas A, Tamary H. Morbidity and mortality of adult patients with congenital dyserythropoietic anemia type I. European Journal of Haematology. 2017;**98**(1):13-18

[15] Fibach E, Rachmilewitz E. Iron overload in hematological disorders. La Presse Médicale. 2017;**46**(12):e296-e305

[16] Ganz T, Nemeth E. Hepcidin and disorders of iron metabolism. Annual Review of Medicine. 2011;**62**:347-360

[17] Rother RP, Bell L, Hillmen P, Gladwin MT. The clinical sequelae of intravascular hemolysis and extracellular plasma hemoglobin—a novel mechanism of human disease. JAMA. 2005;**293**(13):1653-1662

[18] Droge W. Free radicals in the physiological control of cell function. Physiological Reviews. 2002;**82**(1):47-95

[19] Minetti M, Malorni W. Redox control of red blood cell biology: The red blood cell as a target and source of prooxidant species. Antioxidants & Redox Signaling. 2006;**8**(7-8):1165-1169

[20] Mothersill C, Stamato TD, Perez ML, Cummins R, Mooney R, Seymour

CB. Involvement of energy metabolism in the production of 'bystander effects' by radiation. British Journal of Cancer. 2000;**82**(10):1740-1746

[21] Chakraborty A, Held KD, Prise KM, Liber HL, Redmond RW. Bystander effects induced by diffusing mediators after photodynamic stress. Radiation Research. 2009;**172**(1):74-81

[22] Fazi A, Mancini U, Piatti E, Accorsi A, Magnani M. Human red-blood-cells as bioreactors for the inactivation of harmful xenobiotics. Biotechnology and Applied Biochemistry. 1991;**14**(1):60-68

[23] Richards RS, Roberts TK, Dunstan RH, McGregor NR, Butt HL. Erythrocyte antioxidant systems protect cultured endothelial cells against oxidant damage. Biochemistry and Molecular Biology International. 1998;**46**(5):857-865

[24] Richards RS, Roberts TK, McGregor NR, Dunstan RH, Butt HL. The role of erythrocytes in the inactivation of free radicals. Medical Hypotheses. 1998;**50**(5):363-367

[25] Fibach E, Dana M. Oxidative stress: Novel insights on red blood cells as redox modulators. Journal of the International Society of Antioxidants. 2017;**5**(1):10-13

[26] Fibach E, Rachmilewitz EA. The role of antioxidants and iron chelators in the treatment of oxidative stress in thalassemia. Annals of the New York Academy of Sciences. 2010;**1202**:10-16

[27] Ullah A, Khan A, Khan I. Diabetes mellitus and oxidative stress—a concise review. Saudi Pharmaceutical Journal. 2015;**24**(5):547-553

[28] Takahashi MA, Asada K. Superoxide anion permeability of phospholipid-membranes and chloroplast thylakoids. Archives of Biochemistry and Biophysics. 1983;**226**(2):558-566

[29] Lynch RE, Fridovich I. Permeation of erythrocyte stroma by superoxide radical. Journal of Biological Chemistry. 1978;**253**(13):4697-4699

[30] Lavelle F, Puget K, Michelson AM. Function and levels of erythrocupreine in normal humans. Comptes Rendus Hebdomadaires des Seances de l'Academie des Sciences, Serie D. 1974;**278**(21):2695-2698

[31] McCord JM. Free-radicals and inflammation—Protection of synovial-fluid by superoxide-dismutase. Science. 1974;**185**(4150):529-531

[32] Dalmark M. Correction. Journal of Physiology (London). 1972;**226**(2):U289

[33] Buehler PW, Alayash AI. Redox biology of blood revisited: The role of red blood cells in maintaining circulatory reductive capacity. Antioxidants & Redox Signaling. 2005;**7**(11-12):1755-1760

[34] May JM, Qu ZC, Cobb CE. Human erythrocyte recycling of ascorbic acid - relative contributions from the ascorbate free radical and dehydroascorbic acid. Journal of Biological Chemistry. 2004;**279**(15):14975-14982

[35] Freikman I, Amer J, Cohen JS, Ringel I, Fibach E. Oxidative stress causes membrane phospholipid rearrangement and shedding from RBC membranes—An NMR study. Biochimica et Biophysica Acta. 2008;**1778**(10):2388-2394

[36] Ginsburg I, Kohen R, Koren E. Microbial and host cells acquire enhanced oxidant-scavenging abilities by binding polyphenols. Archives of Biochemistry and Biophysics. 2011;**506**(1):12-23

[37] Eldor A, Rachmilewitz EA. The hypercoagulable state in thalassemia. Blood. 2002;**99**(1):36-43

[38] Figueira TR, Barros MH, Camargo AA, Castilho RF, Ferreira JCB, Kowaltowski AJ, et al. Mitochondria as a source of reactive oxygen and nitrogen species: From molecular mechanisms to human health. Antioxidants & Redox Signaling. 2013;**18**(16):2029-2074

[39] Pietraforte D, Vona R, Marchesi A, de Jacobis IT, Villani A, Del Principe D, et al. Redox control of platelet functions in physiology and pathophysiology. Antioxidants & Redox Signaling. 2014;**21**(1):177-193

[40] Seno T, Inoue N, Gao D, Okuda M, Sumi Y, Matsui K, et al. Involvement of NADH/NADPH oxidase in human platelet ROS production. Thrombosis Research. 2001;**103**(5):399-409

[41] Guo LZ, Kim MH, Kim TH, Park JS, Jin EZ, Shim CH, et al. Comparison of three tests to distinguish platelet reactivity in patients with renal impairment during dual antiplatelet therapy. Nephron. 2016;**132**(3):191-197

[42] Hanson SR, Harker LA. Interruption of acute platelet-dependent thrombosis by the synthetic antithrombin D-phenylalanyl-L-prolyl-L-arginyl chloromethyl ketone. Proceedings of the National Academy of Sciences of the United States of America. 1988;**85**(9):3184-3188

[43] Eidt JF, Allison P, Noble S, Ashton J, Golino P, McNatt J, et al. Thrombin is an important mediator of platelet aggregation in stenosed canine coronary arteries with endothelial injury. The Journal of Clinical Investigation. 1989;**84**(1):18-27

[44] Kelly AB, Marzec UM, Krupski W, Bass A, Cadroy Y, Hanson SR, et al. Hirudin interruption of heparin-resistant arterial thrombus formation in baboons. Blood. 1991;**77**(5):1006-1012

[45] Amer J, Fibach E. Oxidative status of platelets in normal and thalassemic blood. Thrombosis and Haemostasis. 2004;**92**(5):1052-1059

[46] Pratico D, Iuliano L, Pulcinelli FM, Bonavita MS, Gazzaniga PP, Violi F. Hydrogen peroxide triggers activation of human platelets selectively exposed to nonaggregating concentrations of arachidonic acid and collagen. The Journal of Laboratory and Clinical Medicine. 1992;**119**(4):364-370

[47] Iuliano L, Colavita AR, Leo R, Pratico D, Violi F. Oxygen free radicals and platelet activation. Free Radical Biology & Medicine. 1997;**22**(6):999-1006

[48] Yamagishi S, Edelstein D, Du XL, Brownlee M. Hyperglycemia potentiates collagen-induced platelet activation through mitochondrial superoxide overproduction. Diabetes. 2001;**50**(6):1491-1494

[49] Krotz F, Sohn HY, Gloe T, Zahler S, Riexinger T, Schiele TM, et al. NAD(P)H oxidase-dependent platelet superoxide anion release increases platelet recruitment. Blood. 2002;**100**(3):917-924

[50] Irani K, Pham Y, Coleman LD, Roos C, Cooke GE, Miodovnik A, et al. Priming of platelet alpha(IIb) beta(3) by oxidants is associated with tyrosine phosphorylation of beta(3). Arteriosclerosis, Thrombosis, and Vascular Biology. 1998;**18**(11):1698-1706

[51] Clutton P, Miermont A, Freedman JE. Regulation of endogenous reactive oxygen species in platelets can reverse aggregation. Arteriosclerosis, Thrombosis, and Vascular Biology. 2004;**24**(1):187-192

[52] Jison ML, Munson PJ, Barb JJ, Suffredini AF, Talwar S, Logun C, et al. Blood mononuclear cell gene expression profiles characterize the oxidant, hemolytic, and inflammatory stress of sickle cell disease. Blood. 2004;**104**(1):270-280

[53] Eldor A. Abnormal platelet functions in beta thalassaemia. Scandinavian Journal of Haematology. 1978;**20**(5):447-452

[54] Amer J, Goldfarb A, Fibach E. Flow cytometric measurement of reactive oxygen species production by normal and thalassaemic red blood cells. European Journal of Haematology. 2003;**70**(2):84-90

[55] Levine PH, Weinger RS, Simon J, Scoon KL, Krinsky NI. Leukocyte-platelet interaction. Release of hydrogen peroxide by granulocytes as a modulator of platelet reactions. The Journal of Clinical Investigation. 1976;**57**(4):955-963

[56] Clark RA, Klebanoff SJ. Neutrophil-platelet interaction mediated by myeloperoxidase and hydrogen peroxide. Journal of Immunology. 1980;**124**(1):399-405

[57] Salvemini D, de Nucci G, Sneddon JM, Vane JR. Superoxide anions enhance platelet adhesion and aggregation. British Journal of Pharmacology. 1989;**97**(4):1145-1150

[58] Iuliano L, Violi F, Pedersen JZ, Pratico D, Rotilio G, Balsano F. Free radical-mediated platelet activation by hemoglobin released from red blood cells. Archives of Biochemistry and Biophysics. 1992;**299**(2):220-224

[59] Thomas MJ. Physiological aspects of low-density lipoprotein oxidation. Current Opinion in Lipidology. 2000;**11**(3):297-301

[60] Malle E, Ibovnik A, Stienmetz A, Kostner GM, Sattler W. Identification of glycoprotein IIb as the lipoprotein(a)-binding protein on platelets. Lipoprotein(a) binding is independent of an arginyl-glycyl-aspartate tripeptide located in apolipoprotein(a). Arteriosclerosis and Thrombosis. 1994;**14**(3):345-352

[61] Solum NO. Procoagulant expression in platelets and defects leading to clinical disorders. Arteriosclerosis, Thrombosis, and Vascular Biology. 1999;**19**(12):2841-2846

[62] Fonseca AM, Porto G, Uchida K, Arosa FA. Red blood cells inhibit activation-induced cell death and oxidative stress in human peripheral blood T lymphocytes. Blood. 2001;**97**(10):3152-3160

[63] Ferro E, Visalli G, Civa R, La Rosa MA, Papa GR, Baluce B, et al. Oxidative damage and genotoxicity biomarkers in transfused and untransfused thalassemic subjects. Free Radical Biology and Medicine. 2012;**53**(10):1829-1837

[64] Ducrocq G, Puymirat E, Steg PG, Henry P, Martelet M, Karam C, et al. Blood transfusion, bleeding, anemia, and survival in patients with acute myocardial infarction: FAST-MI registry. American Heart Journal. 2015;**170**(4):726

[65] Jolicoeur EM, O'Neill WW, Hellkamp A, Hamm CW, Holmes DR, Al-Khalidi HR, et al. Transfusion and mortality in patients with ST-segment elevation myocardial infarction treated with primary percutaneous coronary intervention. European Heart Journal. 2009;**30**(21):2575-2583

[66] Rousseau M, Yan RT, Tan M, Lefkowitz CJ, Casanova A, Fitchett D, et al. Relation between hemoglobin level and recurrent myocardial ischemia in acute coronary syndromes detected by continuous electrocardiographic monitoring. American Journal of Cardiology. 2010;**106**(10):1417-1422

[67] Amer J, Dana M, Fibach E. The antioxidant effect of erythropoietin on thalassemic blood cells. Anemia. 2010;**2010**:978710

[68] Spivak JL. Polycythemia vera. Current Treatment Options in Oncology. 2018;**19**(2):12

[69] Palmer WC, Vishnu P, Sanchez W, Aqel B, Riegert-Johnson D, Seaman LAK, et al. Diagnosis and management of genetic iron overload disorders. Journal of General Internal Medicine. 2018;**33**(12):2230-2236

[70] Amer J, Goldfarb A, Fibach E. Flow cytometric analysis of the oxidative status of normal and thalassemic red blood cells. Cytometry. Part A. 2004;**60**(1):73-80

[71] Prus E, Fibach E. The labile iron pool in human erythroid cells. British Journal of Haematology. 2008;**142**(2):301-307

[72] Bass DA, Parce JW, Dechatelet LR, Szejda P, Seeds MC, Thomas M. Flow cytometric studies of oxidative product formation by neutrophils—A graded response to membrane stimulation. Journal of Immunology. 1983;**130**(4):1910-1917

Chapter 6

Interplay between Erythrocyte Peroxidases and Membrane

Daniela Melo, Susana Rocha, Susana Coimbra and Alice Santos Silva

Abstract

Red blood cells (RBCs) are continuously exposed to oxidative stress (OS), mainly due to their primary function as oxygen carriers. Since RBC is a unique cell, without nucleus or other organelles, it presents a very special metabolism and a highly efficient antioxidant system to face OS conditions. Hemoglobin and RBC membrane are the major targets of oxidative modifications when RBC antioxidant capacity is overwhelmed. Fortunately, non-enzymatic agents, such as glutathione, and enzymatic agents, namely, several peroxidases, such as catalase, glutathione peroxidase and peroxiredoxin 2, are able to prevent OS damage. Although these peroxidases are mainly cytosolic enzymes, evidence exists about their association to the RBC membrane. So far, it appears that the relative importance of the three enzymes is related to hydrogen peroxide levels within the RBC. In this chapter, we will focus on the importance of these peroxidases in the RBC's defense against OS mainly in the RBC cytosol and also the interplay between them and the RBC membrane. The potential role of their binding to the membrane will also be addressed.

Keywords: erythrocyte peroxidases, erythrocyte membrane, hemoglobin, oxidative stress, erythrocyte antioxidant system

1. Introduction

Erythrocytes are the most abundant cells in human blood, with unique morphology and metabolic characteristics and are highly important for body homeostasis. Erythrocytes come from a hematopoietic process—erythropoiesis—by which hematopoietic stem cells from the bone marrow proliferate and differentiate into mature red blood cells (RBCs) [1–3]. Erythrocytes are enucleated cells with a cytoplasm without organelles and rich in hemoglobin (Hb), which represents about 95% of total erythrocyte's cytoplasmic proteins [4, 5].

Membrane structure and composition are responsible for the biconcave disc shape and for the high deformability of the cell. These features are essential for oxygen transport, since RBCs have to undergo repeated shape changes without fragmentation, to assure their passage and oxygen perfusion through all vascular networks, namely, through capillary blood vessels with smaller lumen diameter than that of RBCs [6, 7]. Modifications in RBC membrane protein structure, by decreasing membrane flexibility and stability, may lead to premature removal of the cell reducing RBC's life span [1, 8].

The erythrocyte membrane is a complex structure composed by a lipid bilayer and a protein-based cytoskeleton tethered together by transmembrane proteins, such as protein band 3 and glycophorins. When under oxidative stress (OS) conditions, Hb is oxidized, it binds to the cytoplasmic domain of membrane protein band 3, triggering the formation of aggregates and the covalent linkage of natural anti-band 3 antibodies that may lead to premature RBC removal by splenic macrophages [1, 9].

Hb, the main cytoplasmic protein in RBC, is extremely important for erythrocyte's primary function, as a gas exchanger and for performing oxygen (O_2) distribution to body tissues. Erythrocytes carry O_2 from the lungs to the tissues and mediate carbon dioxide removal from the tissues to the lungs. In the lungs, O_2 binds to the heme group in Hb; in the tissues, O_2 is unloaded from Hb that undergoes a spatial rearrangement of the globin chains, allowing the entry of 2,3-diphosphoglycerate (2,3-DPG) which diminishes O_2 affinity [1, 2]. Oxyhemoglobin suffers autoxidation daily (2–3%), with oxidation of heme ferrous iron into ferric iron [10], leading to the formation of methemoglobin (metHb), which is not capable of O_2 transport, and the release of superoxide anion that is converted to H_2O_2, with a lower oxidant capacity [11]. The erythrocytes are capable of reducing metHb to functional Hb through methemoglobin reductases and of detoxifying the cell from H_2O_2 through the glutathione metabolism [2].

To prevent or reverse the harmful effects of OS, leading to oxidative changes in the erythrocyte constituents, RBCs are equipped with a powerful antioxidant system that is able to protect not only themselves, but also other cells and tissues while circulating throughout the vascular network. The protective antioxidant mechanisms of RBCs include enzymatic and non-enzymatic antioxidant systems that work together to detoxify the cell from reactive oxygen species (ROS) produced within or outside the cell.

In this chapter, we will focus on the importance of the RBC enzymatic antioxidant systems, namely on the peroxidases catalase (CAT), glutathione peroxidase (GPx) and peroxiredoxin 2 (Prx2). These peroxidases have a major role in the RBC's defense against OS, although the interplay between them is still a topic of discussion, as well as the potential role of their binding to the membrane, which may provide a protective mechanism for the cell.

2. Erythrocyte metabolism

Erythrocytes have a limited metabolic capacity since they lack a nucleus and organelles, like mitochondria, for oxidative metabolism [1, 11]. Therefore, energy is generated by the anaerobic glycolytic Embden-Meyerhof pathway, through which the breakdown of glucose to lactate generates two ATP molecules (**Figure 1**). This energy is essential for the maintenance of RBC's shape, membrane deformability and regulation of sodium-potassium pump [1, 2]. This pathway also provides NADH, which is important as a cofactor of methemoglobin reductase to regenerate oxidized Hb to its reduced functional state. The Luebering-Rapoport shunt, a side arm of Embden-Meyerhof pathway, produces 2,3-DPG (**Figure 1**), essential for the regulation of O_2 affinity [1, 2]. Around 80–90% of glucose that enters the cell follows the Embden-Meyerhof pathway, while about 10% is metabolized through the pentose phosphate pathway [12] to ribose-5-phosphate concomitantly generating NADPH (**Figure 1**). NADPH is essential for glutathione (GSH) metabolism that assures the detoxification of RBCs from ROS, being, therefore, an important erythrocyte antioxidant defense mechanism [11].

GSH is a tripeptide constituted by the three amino acids L-glutamate, L-cysteine and L-glycine [13, 14], existing in the cell in two different forms, the reduced form

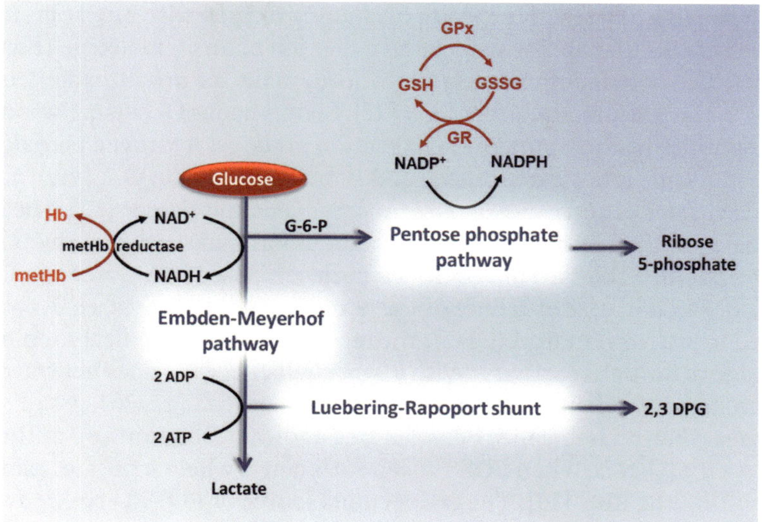

Figure 1.
Erythrocyte metabolic pathways synopsis. 2,3 DPG, 2,3-diphosphoglycerate; ADP, adenosine diphosphate; ATP, adenosine triphosphate; G-6-P, glucose 6-phosphate; GPx, glutathione peroxidase; GR, glutathione reductase; GSSG, oxidized glutathione; GSH, glutathione; Hb, hemoglobin; metHb, methemoglobin; NAD, NADH, nicotinamide adenine dinucleotide; NADP, NADPH, nicotinamide adenine dinucleotide phosphate.

(GSH) and the oxidized form (GSSG). The reduced form is the predominant one and GSSG is maintained at low levels, less than 1% mainly by the action of NADPH-dependent glutathione reductase [13], which converts GSSG into the reduced GSH (**Figure 1**). Despite the limited biosynthesis capability of the RBC, some endogenous GSH is still synthetized in the cytosol through two ATP-dependent reactions catalyzed by two different enzymes, glutamate cysteine ligase and glutathione synthase [13].

As an antioxidant defense, GSH has several roles: it can directly scavenge hydroxyl radicals and peroxynitrites [14, 15]; it is involved in lipid peroxide detoxification [16]; it can reduce H_2O_2 in the presence of GPx by the reduction of its thiol group and keeps thiol groups from Hb, enzymes and membrane proteins in the reduced form [13], which is very important for the preservation of their functions, once oxidation of these groups can lead to functional and structural cellular modifications. Therefore, the GSH/GSSG ratio is an important indicator of the cell redox state [15].

In OS conditions, the capacity of RBCs to reduce GSSG to GSH decreases, leading to GSSG accumulation and, consequently, to GSH depletion [14]. Diminished GSH concentrations have been described in physiological events, as aging, and in pathologic conditions associated with OS, such as Alzheimer's disease, Parkinson's disease [15], sickle cell anemia and asthma [17, 18].

Ascorbic acid (vitamin C) and α-tocopherol (vitamin E) obtained mostly from diet are also important non-enzymatic erythrocyte antioxidants [19]. α-Tocopherol has a protective effect on RBC membranes against lipid peroxidation [11, 19]. Ascorbic acid can reduce O_2^- levels and it is an important regenerator of α-tocopherol. Uric acid can also act as an antioxidant and is able to directly scavenge OH^- [12].

3. Oxidative stress in erythrocytes

During their life span, the erythrocytes are continuously exposed to high O_2 tension, due to their primary function as gas carriers, and are unable to synthesize new or repair damaged proteins, due to the lack of nucleus and other organelles. Therefore, RBCs are more vulnerable to ROS action than other cells of the human body [12].

ROS are chemically reactive species containing oxygen with one or more unpaired electrons that are formed by the reduction of an O_2 molecule (**Figure 2**) [12, 20, 21]. The transfer of one electron to an O_2 molecule produces superoxide anion (O_2^-), the precursor of other ROS [22]. Spontaneous O_2^- dismutation or catalysis by superoxide dismutase (SOD) action produces hydrogen peroxide (H_2O_2) [22]. This molecule is not a free radical and is more stable than O_2^-, but it can easily cross cell membranes and cause damage in other cells and tissues [12]. The RBC needs to be detoxified from H_2O_2, as its accumulation leads to the production of other more potent ROS. This molecule can be decomposed into water and O_2 by CAT, GPx or Prx2. In case of failure of these antioxidant enzymes, H_2O_2 can also be reduced to hydroxyl radical (OH^-), the most harmful free radical for biological systems, due to its high reactivity. With a short half-life, OH^- does not travel far, but has a much higher oxidant potential than all the other ROS [12, 20].

OS arises when an imbalance between free-radical formation and antioxidant defenses occurs, that is, when ROS concentration overwhelms the antioxidant capacity within the RBC [19]. The endogenous source of ROS in erythrocytes is the autoxidation of Hb [11, 12]; occasionally oxyhemoglobin loses one electron (2–3% per day) leading to the production of O_2^- and oxidized Hb (metHb) (**Figure 2**) which is not able to bind and carry O_2. Erythrocytes can also develop OS due to exogenous ROS that are able to diffuse and cross the RBC membrane. The enhanced production and release of ROS by activated inflammatory cells, macrophages, neutrophils and endothelial cells [23], are the main source of exogenous ROS. The continuous exposure of RBCs to ROS can cause cell damage, including lipid and protein oxidation, causing damages in enzymes and ion transport proteins [19, 24].

Considering the major role of Hb, its oxidation may trigger important structural and functional changes in RBCs [11, 12]. Thus, as oxidation of Hb occurs, even under normal physiological conditions, the antioxidant defenses have a crucial role in the regeneration of functional Hb and maintenance of low metHb

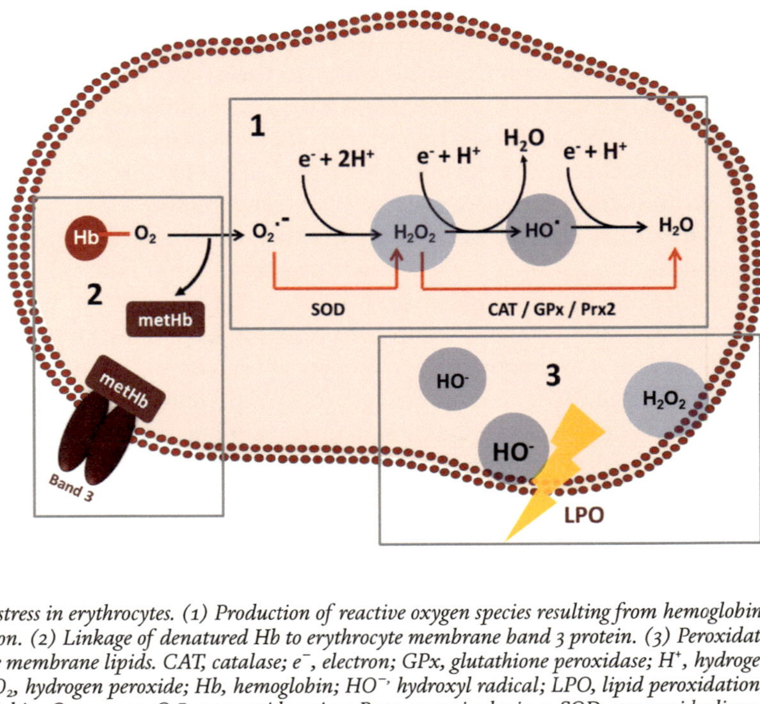

Figure 2.
Oxidative stress in erythrocytes. (1) Production of reactive oxygen species resulting from hemoglobin autoxidation. (2) Linkage of denatured Hb to erythrocyte membrane band 3 protein. (3) Peroxidation of erythrocyte membrane lipids. CAT, catalase; e^-, electron; GPx, glutathione peroxidase; H^+, hydrogen; H_2O, water; H_2O_2, hydrogen peroxide; Hb, hemoglobin; HO^- hydroxyl radical; LPO, lipid peroxidation; metHb, methemoglobin; O_2, oxygen; O_2^-, superoxide anion; Prx2, peroxiredoxin 2; SOD, superoxide dismutase.

levels [11]. When oxidized, the primary structure of Hb is altered by the establishment of disulfide cross-links between globin chains that make the molecule unstable, leading to the formation of Heinz bodies and, eventually, to a premature RBC removal [11]. Indeed, oxidized Hb binds to the cytoplasmic domain of band 3 protein in the RBC membrane (**Figure 2**), triggering band 3 clustering, marking the erythrocyte for removal by splenic macrophages [23, 25]. Clustering of band 3 as a result of enhanced metHb formation and linkage to the membrane has been reported in several erythrocyte disorders such as, hereditary spherocytosis [26], beta-thalassemia [27], sickle cell anemia [28] and glucose-6-phosphate dehydrogenase deficiency [29]. An increase in metHb levels and in its linkage to the RBC membrane, accompanied by ROS formation, was also found in stored RBCs for blood transfusion [30] and in exogenous H_2O_2-induced OS upon healthy erythrocytes [31, 32]. Hb oxidation also occurs as a natural process, resulting from RBC aging [33], that is associated with metabolic degradation due to reduction in enzyme activity.

RBC membrane is an important target for both endogenous and exogenous ROS that may induce oxidative changes in membrane proteins and lipids. Changes in RBC membrane proteins have been reported in some diseases in which OS is involved, such as chronic kidney disease [34, 35] or chronic obstructive pulmonary disease [36]. ROS can affect erythrocyte proteins through oxidation of the protein backbone, cross-linking or amino acid oxidation [19, 24]. The polyunsaturated fatty acids (PUFAs) of the RBC cell membranes are highly vulnerable to oxidation (about half of the RBC membrane fatty acids are unsaturated [12]). ROS are able to break the double bonds of PUFA, producing malondialdehyde (MDA) [24], the main end-product of membrane lipid peroxidation (LPO). MDA is a highly reactive molecule that can further react with lipids and proteins of the membrane. These changes in membrane proteins and lipids contribute to functional and structural alterations that decrease erythrocyte membrane stability and deformability and trigger premature RBC removal [12, 24]. LPO has also been described following metHb binding to the membrane, suggesting that this linkage favors LPO [37]. Increased LPO and MDA levels have been reported in different conditions associated to OS, including physiological events, such as aging [38], and pathological conditions like schizophrenia [39], Alzheimer's disease [40], inflammatory associated diseases [41], atherosclerosis [42] and chronic kidney disease [43]. Considering the reduced biosynthetic capacity of erythrocytes, they accumulate oxidative changes along their life span and, therefore, the OS-induced changes in RBCs could be used as useful biomarkers in several pathological and physiological conditions.

4. Erythrocyte peroxidases

To cope with oxidative injuries, the erythrocytes have several enzymes that neutralize ROS or transform them into less reactive species. SOD provides the first line of protection against free radicals. It is a cytosolic copper-zinc containing enzyme that converts O_2^- into the less reactive H_2O_2 (Eq. (1)), through the alternate reduction and re-oxidation of Cu^{2+} [44].

$$2\,O_2^{\cdot-} + 2H^+ \rightarrow H_2O_2 + O_2 \quad (1)$$

Afterward, H_2O_2 can be decomposed into O_2 and water by three distinct erythrocyte peroxidases: CAT, GPx and Prx2 [45–47].

4.1 Catalase

Catalase (H_2O_2:H_2O_2 oxidoreductase, EC 1.11.1.6) is an intracellular enzyme found at high concentrations in erythrocytes and liver peroxisomes in mammals [48–51]. CAT is a very important enzyme, as it is able to protect cells and tissues from the toxic effects of H_2O_2 [19, 51]. As referred, the decomposition of H_2O_2 is particularly important in erythrocytes, to prevent oxidation of Hb and of other RBC constituents. CAT is one of the most efficient enzymes, since it exhibits one of the fastest turnover rates with a capacity to convert millions of H_2O_2 molecules per second (kcat = $4 \times 10^7\ s^{-1}$) [45, 48].

More than 300 catalase sequences are available, divided among several groups [45, 50, 52]. Human erythrocyte catalase, a tetrameric protein of 244 kDa [53], belongs to the monofunctional heme-containing catalases. Each monomer is formed by a single polypeptide chain that has a molecular weight of approximately 60 kDa [54]. Each subunit also has one heme group at the catalytic center, with iron (III) linked to protoporphyrin IX [53]. Some studies [55–57] showed that each catalase tetramer has four tightly bound NADPH molecules that appear to be important only to protect the enzyme against inactivation by its own substrate (H_2O_2), and are not essential for its catalytic activity. It is thought that NADPH prevents the formation of the inactive form of catalase (Compound II) and that it increases the rate of removal of this inactive form [45, 53, 55, 56].

The overall reaction catalyzed by CAT involves the degradation of two molecules of H_2O_2 to two molecules of water and one of O_2 (Eq. (2)).

$$2\,H_2O_2 \rightarrow 2H_2O + O_2 \tag{2}$$

The H_2O_2 decomposition is believed to occur in two steps (**Figure 3**, steps 1 and 2) [45, 50, 52]. The first involves the interaction between one molecule of H_2O_2 and CAT which leads to the production of Compound I, in which the heme group is oxidized to oxyferryl species [45, 50, 52]. Compound I is an enzymatic active form

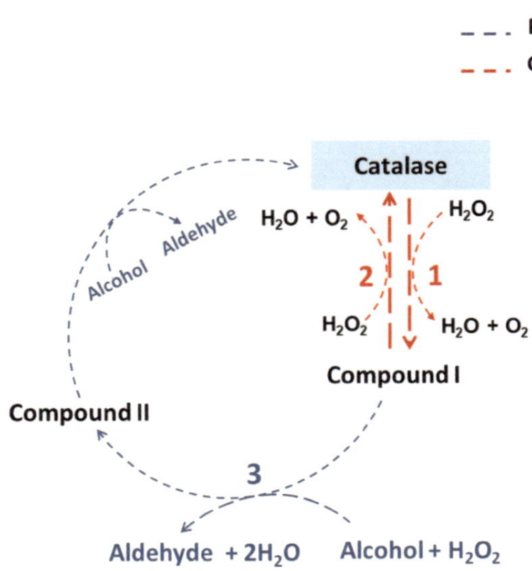

Figure 3.
Hydrogen peroxide removal by catalase. (1) Interaction between H_2O_2 and catalase leading to the production of Compound I. (2) Interaction of a second H_2O_2 molecule with Compound I producing one molecule of H_2O, O_2 and the enzyme at the resting state. (3) Catalase peroxidatic activity. H_2O, water; H_2O_2, hydrogen peroxide; O_2, oxygen.

of catalase but spectroscopically different [58]. At the second step, a second H_2O_2 molecule acts, as a reducing agent, on Compound I, producing one molecule of water, one of O_2 and the enzyme in the resting state [45, 50, 52].

In addition to their catalytic activity, catalases can also function peroxidatively (**Figure 3**, step 3) to eliminate H_2O_2 [45, 49]. In this case, the enzyme uses peroxidation to eliminate H_2O_2 molecules by oxidizing substances like alcohols. The peroxidatic activity of CAT is, usually, minor, weak and restricted to smaller substrates, as compared to other peroxidases [45].

When compared with the other H_2O_2 scavenger enzymes, CAT seems to be the key enzyme to remove high intracellular concentrations of H_2O_2 [32, 53, 59, 60]. Moreover, CAT is highly specific for its substrate, H_2O_2, and it is not able to eliminate organic peroxides, unlike other peroxidases [59].

Catalase has also been studied in a number of different diseases in which OS is implicated, such as, diabetes mellitus where patients presented lower CAT values [61]; in some type of cancers, CAT activity was lower in patients, especially in lymphomas, when compared with CAT activity in the normal population [62] and, in bipolar disorder, subjects with bipolar depression presented a significant increase in CAT levels [63].

4.2 Glutathione peroxidase

GPx (GSH_2:H_2O_2 oxidoreductase, EC 1.11.1.9) is an intracellular antioxidant enzyme that contributes to prevent H_2O_2 accumulation in cells. In mammals, eight GPxs have been identified [47] at different locations and cellular compartments, differing at their catalytic center. GPx-1 is one of the most abundant type of GPx and the only type present in RBC's cytosol [60]. GPx-1 is a tetramer of four identical subunits of 21 kDa [64], each with one selenocysteine (Sec) [65]. The catalytic tetrad formed by Sec, glutamine, tryptophan and asparagine is essential for GPx activity, since these residues are crucial for enzyme-substrate interaction and stabilization of the GSH-GPx interaction [47, 65, 66].

GPx-1 catalyzes the reduction of H_2O_2 [47, 66], lipid hydroperoxides and other low molecular hydroperoxides [64] into water, or into the corresponding alcohols, using GSH as a reducing agent; thus, GPx-1 prevents both lipid peroxidation [65, 67] and H_2O_2 accumulation.

The overall catalytic reaction of GPx-1 is given by Eq. (3).

$$ROOH + 2GSH \rightarrow ROH + H_2O + GSSG \qquad (3)$$

The catalytic cycle of GPx includes a peroxidatic part that is followed by a reductive step (**Figure 4**) [47]. In the peroxidatic part, one molecule of H_2O_2 reacts with the selenol group from Sec in GPx, producing a selenenic acid at the active site [47, 66]. In the reductive part, one GSH molecule forms a selenadisulfide bond with the selenic acid forming the glutathiolated selenol intermediate [47]. As a second GSH molecule reduces the glutathiolated selenol bond, GSSG is released and GPx is regenerated. The restoration of GSH involves the action of the NADPH-dependent enzyme, glutathione reductase. The recycling of NADPH associates the GSH system to the pentose-phosphate pathway [66].

CAT was considered as the only enzyme involved in erythrocyte antioxidant defense by performing H_2O_2 removal [68]. Nowadays, it is known that GPx also has a major role in RBC antioxidant protection, being essential for the detoxification of low H_2O_2 concentrations and hydroperoxides [59, 69, 70], with a constant rate superior to $10^7\ M^{-1}\ s^{-1}$ [47, 71].

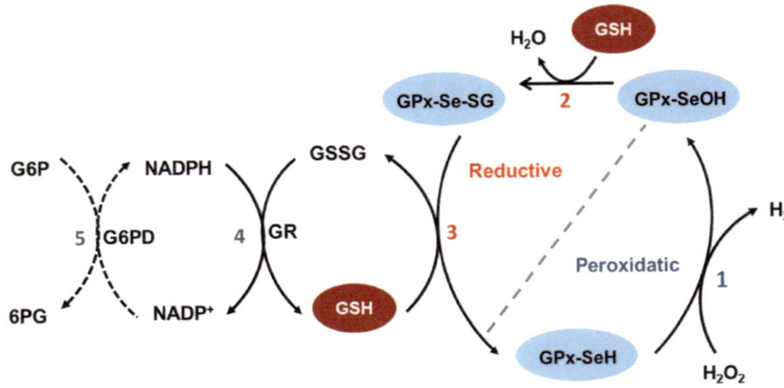

Figure 4.
Catalytic cycle of glutathione peroxidase 1. (1) Peroxidatic part of GPx-1 catalytic cycle. (2) and (3) Reductive part of GPx-1 catalytic cycle (4) Regeneration of GSH by NADPH-dependent GR. (5) $NADP^+$/NADPH recycling by G6PD. 6PG, 6-phosphogluconolactone; G6P, glucose-6-phosphate; G6PD, glucose-6-phosphate dehydrogenase; GPx-SeH, glutathione peroxidase selenol; GPx-SeOH, glutathione peroxidase selenic acid; GPx-Se-SG, glutathiolated selenol intermediate; GR, glutathione reductase; GSH, glutathione; GSSG, oxidized glutathione; H_2O, water; H_2O_2, hydrogen peroxide; NADPH/$NADP^+$, nicotinamide adenine dinucleotide phosphate.

4.3 Peroxiredoxin 2

Peroxiredoxins (Prxs; SH:H_2O_2 oxidoreductases, EC 1.11.1.15) are a family of homodimeric peroxidases with an antioxidant role in living organisms. Six different mammalian Prx isoforms are known (Prx 1–6). Prx 1 and Prx 6 can be found in erythrocytes, although in much lower amounts than Prx2, which is the third most abundant protein in the RBC cytosol (after Hb and carbonic anhydrase) [5].

For a long time, CAT and GPx were considered the major erythrocyte players for H_2O_2 detoxification [68]. However, several studies [72–75] have shown the significant role of Prx2 as an efficient H_2O_2 scavenger in the erythrocyte antioxidant system. Studies using Prx2 knock-out mice showed that these animal models developed hemolytic anemia and their erythrocytes displayed a significantly shorter life span, when compared to wild-type mice [72]. In contrast, CAT and GPx knock-out mice showed a normal hematologic profile and normal development [72, 76]. Another important study reported that Prx2 reacts with H_2O_2 at a constant rate ($1.3 \times 10^7\ M^{-1}\ s^{-1}$) comparable with that of CAT and GPx [75].

Under its physiological functional state, Prx2 appears as a monomer (active form) of about 20–30 kDa and when interacting with H_2O_2, Prx2 is oxidized and a disulfide-linked dimmer is formed (inactive form) [73, 77]. This oxidized form is reversed by thioredoxin (Trx)/Trx reductase/NADPH system, although, in RBCs, it is a very slow regeneration due to the low concentrations of Trx reductase [73]. Besides H_2O_2, Prx2 can also remove peroxynitrites [5] and hydroperoxides in the RBC membrane [73, 75].

Since Prx2 is a thiol-dependent peroxidase, it uses redox-active cysteines to reduce peroxides. According to the number and location of the catalytic cysteines, Prxs are divided into three classes: the typical 2-Cys, the atypical 2-Cys and the 1-Cys [46]. Prx2 is a typical 2-Cys peroxiredoxin, with two redox-active cysteines: the peroxidatic cysteine near residue 50 in one subunit and the resolving cysteine near residue 170 in the other subunit [46]. The overall peroxidase reaction is given by Eq. (4).

$$\mathbf{ROOH + 2e^- \rightarrow ROH + H_2O} \tag{4}$$

The catalytic cycle of Prx2 is composed by two steps (**Figure 5**). The first step is the oxidation of peroxidatic cysteine to peroxidatic cysteine-sulfenic acid by interaction with H_2O_2. In the second step, the resolving cysteine of one Prx subunit attacks the peroxidatic cysteine-sulfenic acid of the other subunit generating an inter-subunit disulfide bond [46, 75]. This dimeric form of Prx2 is non-functional, but the disulfide bridge between the subunits can be broken by Trx, regenerating Prx2, and completing the catalytic cycle [73]. In turn, Trx can be reduced by the NADPH-dependent Trx reductase. Reduction of the disulfide bond by Trx is the rate-limiting step in the Prx2 catalytic cycle [73].

In the presence of high peroxide levels, 2-Cys Prxs can become over-oxidized to their sulfinic acid form. In RBCs, this hyperoxidation of Prx2 does not occur, as it is counteracted by sulfiredoxin [60, 73].

As part of the erythrocyte antioxidant system, Prx2 is responsible for the removal of low H_2O_2 concentrations, since the Trx system has a limited capacity for Prx2 regeneration into its reduced active form [32, 59, 60, 73]. Recently, it was found that Prx2 can have a dual function according to H_2O_2 levels, as an antioxidant enzyme or as a chaperone, due to changes in its structure [59, 73, 78]. In RBCs, Prx2 can bind to Hb under OS conditions to stabilize its structure and prevent Hb aggregation [79]. A recent work by our group [80] showed that under steady-state conditions, Prx2 acts as a typical peroxidase, protecting the erythrocytes from low endogenous levels of ROS. However, when RBCs are saturated with carbon monoxide, Prx2 was observed only in the active form in the cytosol and none in the oxidized form, suggesting that Prx2 is acting specifically to protect Hb, shifting its function from peroxidase to chaperone. Prx2, initially called calpromotin, is also required to regulate the calcium-dependent potassium channel in the erythrocyte membrane [81].

The use of Prx2 as a potential therapeutic drug target has gained growing interest; so far, it has already been reported as a possible target for malaria treatment [82]. Changes in human Prx2 expression or oxidation state have been associated with several diseases: alterations in Prx2 expression have been reported in different types of cancer [83, 84]; oxidatively modified Prx2 has been found in Alzheimer's disease patients [85]; hyperoxidized forms of Prx2 were also found in asthmatic patients [86] and linkage of cytosolic Prx2 to the RBC membrane was found in

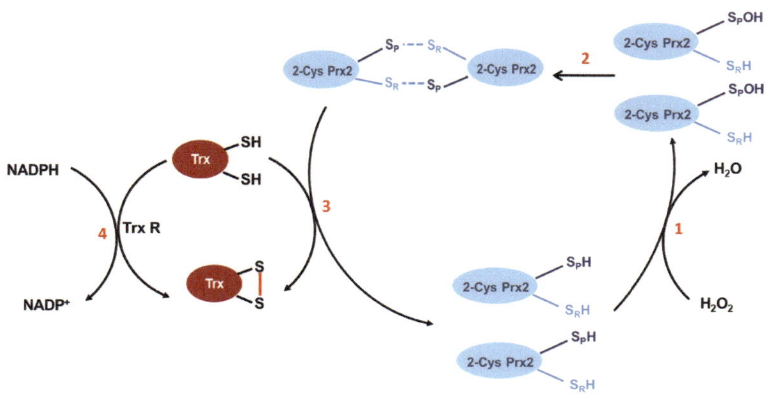

Figure 5.
Peroxiredoxin 2 catalytic cycle. (1) Oxidation of S_PH to S_POH by interaction with H_2O_2. (2) Attack of S_RH of one subunit to S_POH of the other subunit and formation of the intersubunit disulfide bond. (3) Reduction of the disulfide bond by Trx. (4) Regeneration of reduced Trx by NADPH-dependent Trx reductase. 2-Cys Prx, 2-cys peroxiredoxin 2; H_2O, water; H_2O_2, hydrogen peroxide; NADPH/NADP$^+$, nicotinamide adenine dinucleotide phosphate; S_PH, peroxidatic cysteine; S_POH, peroxidatic cysteine sulfenic acid; S_RH, resolving cysteine; Trx, thioredoxin; TrxR, thioredoxin reductase.

hereditary spherocytosis patients [26]. Thus, there has been an increasing interest in Prx2 as a biomarker for different conditions where OS plays a crucial role. For example, a novel HPLC method to monitor the levels of reduced Prx2 form was developed [87], which could prove useful for future clinical practice.

5. Interplay between erythrocyte peroxidases and the erythrocyte membrane

The individual contribution of CAT, GPx and Prx2 to erythrocyte protection against H_2O_2 damage has been a controversial issue for many years. It is clear that all three enzymes are involved in the prevention of H_2O_2 accumulation in the RBC through H_2O_2 conversion into water and O_2 (**Figure 6**); however, the relative importance of the three enzymes is still a topic of discussion.

CAT was considered the main erythrocyte defense against OS, for many years [68, 88], but several studies [59, 69, 89] showed that GPx has also an important role in H_2O_2 decomposition. In fact, a study by Johnson et al. [59] showed that CAT and GPx-deficient RBCs were more sensitive to H_2O_2-induced OS than cells with only CAT deficiency, suggesting that GPx has an important role in erythrocyte defense. The same authors also showed [59, 70] that the action of both CAT and GPx was insufficient to explain the erythrocyte oxidative catabolism, and proposed [70] a model including Prx2 that, in accordance with their experimental data, could better explain the erythrocyte antioxidant defense system. Furthermore, the development of hemolytic anemia in Prx2 knock-out mice [72–74] and the high turnover rate of Prx2 with H_2O_2 [5, 75] strengthened the importance of the role of Prx2 in RBC antioxidant protection.

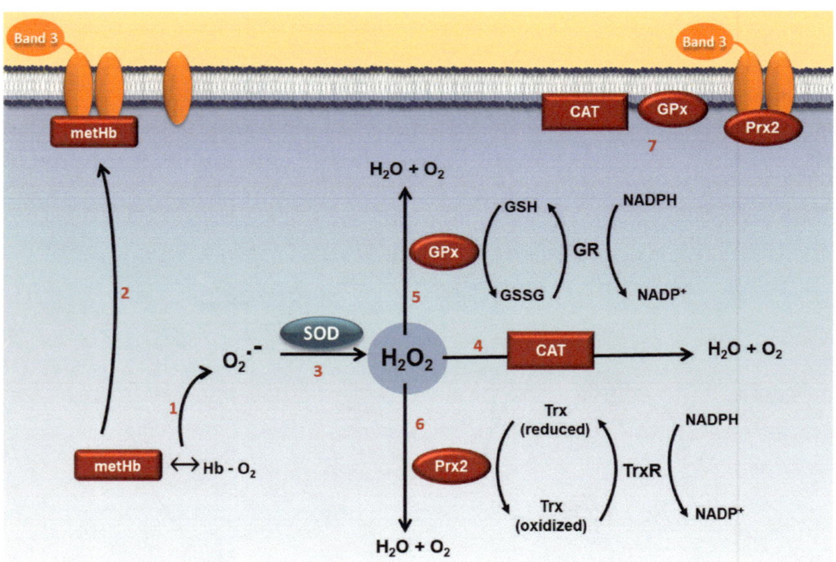

Figure 6.
Interplay between erythrocyte's peroxidases. (1) Methemoglobin formation and release of O_2^{-}. (2) Formation of band 3 protein aggregates triggered by methemoglobin linkage to the integral membrane protein band 3. (3) O_2^{-} removal by SOD with H_2O_2 formation. (4) H_2O_2 removal by CAT. (5) H_2O_2 removal by GPx. (6) H_2O_2 removal by Prx2. (7) Linkage of CAT, GPx and Prx2 to the RBC membrane imposed by oxidative stress. CAT, catalase; GPx, glutathione peroxidase; GR, glutathione reductase; GSH, glutathione; GSSG, oxidized glutathione; H_2O, water; H_2O_2, hydrogen peroxide; Hb, hemoglobin; metHb, methemoglobin; Hb-O_2, oxyhemoglobin; NADPH/NADP$^+$, nicotinamide adenine dinucleotide phosphate; O2, oxygen; O_2^{-}, superoxide anion; Prx2, peroxiredoxin 2; SOD, superoxide dismutase; Trx, thioredoxin; TrxR, thioredoxin reductase.

The relative importance of the three enzymes appears to be related to the H_2O_2 levels in the RBC [59]. CAT is able to scavenge exogenous and high endogenous peroxide levels [59, 60, 70], while GPx and Prx2 appear to scavenge endogenous and low peroxide levels [59, 70, 73]. Thus, the elimination of the basal flux and low H_2O_2 levels is performed by GPx and Prx2, since CAT does not work efficiently at low H_2O_2 levels [60]. Whenever RBCs are exposed to higher H_2O_2 levels, CAT becomes essential for its rapid removal since this enzyme has a high turnover rate, unlike GPx and Prx2 that become less efficient (or even inactive), due to their slow GSH reductase and Trx recycling systems, respectively [59, 60, 73].

The enzymes GPx and Prx2 seem to have other functions in RBC antioxidant defense, beyond H_2O_2 scavenging. In fact, GPx and Prx2 are also able to detoxify organic peroxides [5, 59, 75], while CAT does not show this function [59]. As shown by Johnson et al. [59, 90], GPx-deficient RBCs are more susceptible to oxidation by organic peroxides than wild type cells [90]; and when CAT deficiency was added to GPx deficiency, no increased sensitivity to oxidation by organic peroxides occurred in these cells [59]. Thus, when erythrocytes are exposed to high H_2O_2 levels, organic peroxides will accumulate, since GPx and Prx2 become less efficient and CAT is not able to detoxify these organic peroxides [60].

Recently, it was reported that Prx2 can have multiple functions, as a peroxidase or as a chaperone, through the formation of high-molecular-weight complexes [78, 91]. It was shown that Prx2 acts as a chaperone in RBCs, by interacting directly with Hb to maintain its stability [79]. A study by our group [80] showed that when erythrocytes were saturated with CO, the enzyme Prx2 was present in the cytosol only in the monomeric form, suggesting that Prx2 was not acting as a peroxidase but, instead, exclusively as a chaperone for Hb's protection. Several authors have suggested [59, 92] that Prx2 can also have an important role in erythropoiesis. Johnson et al. [59] believe that the role of Prx2 as Hb chaperone is especially important in the different stages of erythropoiesis. According to Matte et al., Prx2 appears to be a regulator of iron homeostasis during erythropoiesis [92].

CAT, GPx and Prx2 are essentially cytosolic enzymes; however, the association of these enzymes to the erythrocyte membrane has been reported in different in vivo and in vitro studies [26, 31, 32, 93–97]. Erythrocytes from patients with hereditary spherocytosis showed CAT [95] and Prx2 bound to their membranes [26]. The association of CAT to the membrane appears to be a consequence of the metabolic stress triggered by the destabilization of membrane structure, due to an altered RBC membrane composition; the linkage of Prx2 might be involved in the protection of the RBC membrane against LPO [26, 31]. This linkage of Prx2 to the membrane appears to be through the N-terminal cytoplasmic domain of band 3, which is also the site of linkage of other cytoplasmic proteins, including metHb [98]. In recent in vitro assays performed by our group [32], we showed that H_2O_2-induced oxidative stress triggered the binding of Prx2 and GPx to RBC membrane. A recent study by Bayer et al. [96] about the interaction of Prx2 with the RBC membrane reported that the linkage of Prx2 to the membrane is independent of its redox state and that Prx2 competes with Hb for the same binding site in the RBC membrane. Thus, they demonstrated that Prx2 prevents metHb aggregation, and, probably acts as a chaperone for the denatured Hb [96]. Contrary to what was previously observed [26, 31, 32], Bayer et al. [96] found a decrease in Prx2 membrane binding, with increasing concentrations of H_2O_2. A decrease in Prx2 linkage to the RBC membrane with OS conditions was also observed in beta-thalassemic mice RBCs, probably due to the increase in metHb that binds to the membrane, reducing the access of Prx2 to the same site [99].

The linkage of GPx to the RBC membrane was first described by van Gestel et al., using proteome analysis [94]. Later on, Rocha et al. showed the linkage of GPx to the RBC membrane in response to in vitro H_2O_2-induced OS [32].

Studies of stored RBCs in blood bank conditions also reported the recruitment of Prx2, CAT and GPx to the RBC membrane due to OS modifications resulting from the metabolic stress of long-term erythrocyte storage [93, 97].

Data in literature suggest that the linkage of these RBC cytosolic enzymes to the membrane is triggered by metabolic stress, possibly, to protect the erythrocyte membrane and counteract the effects of OS.

6. Conclusions

Erythrocytes, as oxygen carrier cells, are highly exposed to oxidative injury; to face this challenge, RBCs are well equipped with an efficient antioxidant system, important to maintain erythrocyte homeostasis during its life span. The antioxidant system includes non-enzymatic and enzymatic agents such as peroxidases, namely Prx2, GPx and CAT. The role and interplay between these enzymes that prevent H_2O_2 accumulation in the erythrocyte has been a topic of discussion over the years. So far, it appears that their role depends on the H_2O_2 levels within RBC: CAT is crucial for scavenging high exogenous and endogenous peroxide levels, GPx and Prx2 are important for scavenging low endogenous and low peroxide levels. GPx and Prx2 are also able to detoxify the cell from organic peroxides, unlike CAT that does not show this function. Therefore, GPx and Prx2 can have a direct role on RBC membrane antioxidant defense.

Several authors have already reported the linkage of CAT, GPx and Prx2 to the erythrocyte membrane in case of metabolic stress and/or OS. In fact, the recruitment of the three peroxidases to the RBC membrane has been described in OS-associated conditions, by in vitro assays and by studies with stored RBCs under blood bank conditions.

Studies about Prx2 reveal a dual function in RBC defense, as a peroxidase and as an Hb chaperone preventing metHb aggregation. Some authors have also proposed that Prx2 may have a major role in erythropoiesis.

Erythrocytes are the ultimate antioxidant defense against the harmful effects of OS in humans; so, the knowledge about the RBC antioxidant system has evolved over time, and should continue to grow, focusing on the importance of CAT, GPx and Prx2 working together in ROS detoxification and also their potential role in the erythrocyte membrane.

Acknowledgements

Financial support from FCT/MCTES through national funds UID/MULTI/04378/2019 and Norte Portugal Regional Coordination and Development Commission (CCDR-N)/NORTE2020/Portugal 2020 (Norte-01-0145-FEDER-000024) and a PhD grant (SRRH/BD/139622/2018) attributed to D. Melo.

Conflict of interest

The authors report no conflict of interest.

Author details

Daniela Melo[1], Susana Rocha[1], Susana Coimbra[2,3] and Alice Santos Silva[1]*

1 UCIBIO, REQUIMTE, Laboratory of Biochemistry, Department of Biological Sciences, Faculty of Pharmacy, University of Porto, Porto, Portugal

2 UCIBIO, REQUIMTE, Porto, Portugal

3 CESPU, Institute of research and Advanced Training in Health Sciences and Technologies (IINFACTS), Gandra-Paredes, Portugal

*Address all correspondence to: assilva@ff.up.pt

References

[1] Turgeon ML. Clinical Hematology: Theory and Procedures. 5th ed. USA: Lippincott Williams & Wilkins; 2010

[2] Hoffbrand AV, Moss PAH, Pettit IE. Essential Haematology. 5th ed. USA: Blackwell Publishing Ltd; 2006

[3] Tsiftsoglou AS, Vizirianakis IS, Strouboulis J. Erythropoiesis: Model systems, molecular regulators, and developmental programs. IUBMB Life. 2009;**61**(8):800-830. DOI: 10.1002/iub.226

[4] Hattangadi SM et al. From stem cell to red cell: Regulation of erythropoiesis at multiple levels by multiple proteins, RNAs, and chromatin modifications. Blood. 2011;**118**(24):6258-6268. DOI: 10.1182/blood-2011-07-356006

[5] Manta B et al. The peroxidase and peroxynitrite reductase activity of human erythrocyte peroxiredoxin 2. Archives of Biochemistry and Biophysics. 2009;**484**(2):146-154. DOI: 10.1016/j.abb.2008.11.017

[6] Diez-Silva M et al. Shape and biomechanical characteristics of human red blood cells in health and disease. MRS Bulletin. 2010;**35**(5):382-388

[7] Mohandas N. Molecular basis for red cell membrane viscoelastic properties. Biochemical Society Transactions. 1992;**20**(4):776-782. DOI: 10.1042/bst0200776

[8] An X, Mohandas N. Disorders of red cell membrane. British Journal of Haematology. 2008;**141**(3):367-375. DOI: 10.1111/j.1365-2141.2008.07091.x

[9] Kay MM, Wyant T, Goodman J. Autoantibodies to band 3 during aging and disease and aging interventions. Annals of the New York Academy of Sciences. 1994;**719**:419-447. DOI: 10.1111/j.1749-6632.1994.tb56847.x

[10] Umbreit J. Methemoglobin-it's not just blue: A concise review. American Journal of Hematology. 2007;**82**(2):134-144. DOI: 10.1002/ajh.20738

[11] Pandey KB, Rizvi SI. Biomarkers of oxidative stress in red blood cells. Biomedical Papers. 2011;**155**(2):131-136. DOI: 10.5507/bp.2011.027

[12] Çimen MYB. Free radical metabolism in human erythrocytes. Clinica Chimica Acta. 2008;**390**(1-2):1-11. DOI: 10.1016/j.cca.2007.12.025

[13] Lu SC. Regulation of glutathione synthesis. Molecular Aspects of Medicine. 2009;**30**(1-2):42-59. DOI: 10.1016/j.mam.2008.05.005

[14] Griffith OW. Biologic and pharmacologic regulation of mammalian glutathione synthesis. Free Radical Biology & Medicine. 1999;**27**(9-10):922-935. DOI: 10.1016/S0891-5849(99)00176-8

[15] Wu G et al. Glutathione metabolism and its implications for health. The Journal of Nutrition. 2004;**134**(3):489-492. DOI: 10.1093/jn/134.3.489

[16] Raftos JE, Whillier S, Kuchel PW. Glutathione synthesis and turnover in the human erythrocyte: Alignment of a model based on detailed enzyme kinetics with experimental data. The Journal of Biological Chemistry. 2010;**285**(31):23557-23567. DOI: 10.1074/jbc.M109.067017

[17] Pace BS et al. Effects of N-acetylcysteine on dense cell formation in sickle cell disease. American Journal of Hematology. 2003;**73**(1):26-32. DOI: 10.1002/ajh.10321

[18] Fitzpatrick AM, Jones DP, Brown LAS. Glutathione redox control of asthma: From molecular mechanisms to therapeutic opportunities. Antioxidants

& Redox Signaling. 2012;**17**(2):375-408. DOI: 10.1089/ars.2011.4198

[19] Lobo V et al. Free radicals, antioxidants and functional foods: Impact on human health. Pharmacognosy Reviews. 2010;**4**(8):118-126. DOI: 10.4103/0973-7847.70902

[20] Valko M et al. Free radicals and antioxidants in normal physiological functions and human disease. The International Journal of Biochemistry & Cell Biology. 2007;**39**(1):44-84. DOI: 10.1016/j.biocel.2006.07.001

[21] Fridovich I. Oxygen: How do we stand it? Medical Principles and Practice. 2013;**22**(2):131-137. DOI: 10.1159/000339212

[22] Turrens JF. Mitochondrial formation of reactive oxygen species. The Journal of Physiology. 2003;**552**(Pt 2):335-344. DOI: 10.1113/jphysiol.2003.049478

[23] Mohanty JG, Nagababu E, Rifkind JM. Red blood cell oxidative stress impairs oxygen delivery and induces red blood cell aging. Frontiers in Physiology. 2014;**5**:84. 1-6. DOI: 10.3389/fphys.2014.00084

[24] Maurya PK, Kumar P, Chandra P. Biomarkers of oxidative stress in erythrocytes as a function of human age. World Journal of Methodology. 2015;**5**(4):216-222. DOI: 10.5662/wjm.v5.i4.216

[25] Arashiki N et al. Membrane peroxidation and methemoglobin formation are both necessary for band 3 clustering: Mechanistic insights into human erythrocyte senescence. Biochemistry. 2013;**52**(34):5760-5769. DOI: 10.1021/bi400405p

[26] Rocha S et al. Presence of cytosolic peroxiredoxin 2 in the erythrocyte membrane of patients with hereditary spherocytosis. Blood Cells, Molecules & Diseases. 2008;**41**(1):5-9. DOI: 10.1016/j.bcmd.2008.02.008

[27] Mannu F et al. Role of hemichrome binding to erythrocyte membrane in the generation of band-3 alterations in beta-thalassemia intermedia erythrocytes. Blood. 1995;**86**(5):2014-2020

[28] Waugh SM et al. Heinz bodies induce clustering of band 3, glycophorin, and ankyrin in sickle cell erythrocytes. The Journal of Clinical Investigation. 1986;**78**(5):1155-1160. DOI: 10.1172/JCI112696

[29] Pantaleo A et al. Oxidized and poorly glycosylated band 3 is selectively phosphorylated by Syk kinase to form large membrane clusters in normal and G6PD-deficient red blood cells. The Biochemical Journal. 2009;**418**(2):359-367. DOI: 10.1042/BJ20081557

[30] Kanias T, Acker JP. Biopreservation of red blood cells--the struggle with hemoglobin oxidation. The FEBS Journal. 2010;**277**(2):343-356. DOI: 10.1111/j.1742-4658.2009.07472.x

[31] Rocha S et al. Linkage of cytosolic peroxiredoxin 2 to erythrocyte membrane imposed by hydrogen peroxide-induced oxidative stress. Blood Cells, Molecules & Diseases. 2009;**43**(1):68-73. DOI: 10.1016/j.bcmd.2009.03.002

[32] Rocha S et al. Peroxiredoxin 2, glutathione peroxidase, and catalase in the cytosol and membrane of erythrocytes under H_2O_2-induced oxidative stress. Free Radical Research. 2015;**49**(8):990-1003. DOI: 10.3109/10715762.2015.1028402

[33] Low PS et al. The role of hemoglobin denaturation and band 3 clustering in red blood cell aging. Science. 1985;**227**(4686):531-533. DOI: 10.1126/science.2578228

[34] Costa E et al. Altered erythrocyte membrane protein composition in

chronic kidney disease stage 5 patients under haemodialysis and recombinant human erythropoietin therapy. Blood Purification. 2008;**26**(3):267-273. DOI: 10.1159/000126922

[35] Costa E et al. Changes in red blood cells membrane protein composition during hemodialysis procedure. Renal Failure. 2008;**30**(10):971-975. DOI: 10.1080/08860220802422036

[36] Torres-Ramos YD et al. RBC membrane damage and decreased band 3 phospho-tyrosine phosphatase activity are markers of COPD progression. Frontiers in Bioscience (Elite Edition). 2010;**2**:1385-1393

[37] Kanner J, Harel S. Initiation of membranal lipid peroxidation by activated metmyoglobin and methemoglobin. Archives of Biochemistry and Biophysics. 1985;**237**(2):314-321. DOI: 10.1016/0003-9861(85)90282-6

[38] Pandey KB, Rizvi SI. Markers of oxidative stress in erythrocytes and plasma during aging in humans. Oxidative Medicine and Cellular Longevity. 2010;**3**(1):2-12. DOI: 10.4161/oxim.3.1.10476

[39] Altuntas I et al. Erythrocyte superoxide dismutase and glutathione peroxidase activities, and malondialdehyde and reduced glutathione levels in schizophrenic patients. Clinical Chemistry and Laboratory Medicine. 2000;**38**(12):1277-1281. DOI: 10.1515/CCLM.2000.201

[40] Lovell MA et al. Elevated thiobarbituric acid-reactive substances and antioxidant enzyme activity in the brain in Alzheimer's disease. Neurology. 1995;**45**(8):1594-1601. DOI: 10.1212/WNL.45.8.1594

[41] Leitinger N. The role of phospholipid oxidation products in inflammatory and autoimmune diseases: Evidence from animal models and in humans. Subcellular Biochemistry. 2008;**49**:325-350. DOI: 10.1007/978-1-4020-8830-8_12

[42] Lee S et al. Role of phospholipid oxidation products in atherosclerosis. Circulation Research. 2012;**111**(6): 778-799. DOI: 10.1161/CIRCRESAHA.111.256859

[43] Durak İ et al. Oxidant/antioxidant status of erythrocytes from patients with chronic renal failure: Effects of hemodialysis. Medical Principles and Practice. 2001;**10**(4):187-190. DOI: 10.1159/000050367

[44] Mondola P et al. The Cu, Zn superoxide dismutase: Not only a dismutase enzyme. Frontiers in Physiology. 2016;**7**:594. 1-8. DOI: 10.3389/fphys.2016.00594

[45] Nicholls P, Peter C. Enzymology and structure of catalases. Advances in Inorganic Chemistry. 2000;**51**:51-106. DOI: 10.1016/S0898-8838(00)51001-0

[46] Wood ZA et al. Structure, mechanism and regulation of peroxiredoxins. Trends in Biochemical Sciences. 2003;**28**(1):32-40. DOI: 10.1016/S0968-0004(02)00003-8

[47] Brigelius-Flohe R, Maiorino M. Glutathione peroxidases. Biochimica et Biophysica Acta. 2013;**1830**(5):3289-3303. DOI: 10.1016/j.bbagen.2012.11.020

[48] Berg JM, Tymoczko JL, Stryer L. Biochemistry. 5th ed. USA: W.H. Freeman; 2002

[49] Yasemin BM, Hamdi O, Nazmi O. The mechanism of inhibition of human erythrocyte catalase by azide. Turkish Journal of Biology. 2004;**28**:65-70

[50] Switala J, Loewen PC. Diversity of properties among catalases. Archives

of Biochemistry and Biophysics. 2002;**401**(2):145-154. DOI: 10.1007/s00018-003-3206-5

[51] Reid TJ et al. Structure and heme environment of beef liver catalase at 2.5 A resolution. Proceedings of the National Academy of Sciences of the United States of America. 1981;**78**(8):4767-4771. DOI: 10.1073/pnas.78.8.4767

[52] Chelikani P, Fita I, Loewen PC. Diversity of structures and properties among catalases. Cellular and Molecular Life Sciences. 2004;**61**(2):192-208. DOI: 10.1007/s00018-003-3206-5

[53] Kodydkova J et al. Human catalase, its polymorphisms, regulation and changes of its activity in different diseases. Folia Biologica (Praha). 2014;**60**(4):153-167

[54] Vainshtein BK et al. Three-dimensional structure of the enzyme catalase. Nature. 1981;**293**(5831):411-412

[55] Kirkman HN et al. Mechanisms of protection of catalase by NADPH. Kinetics and stoichiometry. The Journal of Biological Chemistry. 1999;**274**(20):13908-13914. DOI: 10.1074/jbc.274.20.13908

[56] Kirkman HN, Galiano S, Gaetani GF. The function of catalase-bound NADPH. The Journal of Biological Chemistry. 1987;**262**(2):660-666

[57] Kirkman HN, Gaetani GF. Catalase: A tetrameric enzyme with four tightly bound molecules of NADPH. Proceedings of the National Academy of Sciences of the United States of America. 1984;**81**(14):4343-4347. DOI: 10.1073/pnas.81.14.4343

[58] Chance B. An intermediate compound in the catalase-hydrogen peroxide reaction. Acta Chemica Scandinavica. 1947;**1**:236-267. DOI: 10.3891/acta.chem.scand.01-0236

[59] Johnson RM et al. The effects of disruption of genes for peroxiredoxin-2, glutathione peroxidase-1, and catalase on erythrocyte oxidative metabolism. Free Radical Biology & Medicine. 2010;**48**(4):519-525. DOI: 10.1016/j.freeradbiomed.2009.11.021

[60] Cho CS et al. Irreversible inactivation of glutathione peroxidase 1 and reversible inactivation of peroxiredoxin II by H_2O_2 in red blood cells. Antioxidants & Redox Signaling. 2010;**12**(11):1235-1246. DOI: 10.1089/ars.2009.2701

[61] Abou-Seif MA, Youssef AA. Evaluation of some biochemical changes in diabetic patients. Clinica Chimica Acta. 2004;**346**(2):161-170. DOI: 10.1016/j.cccn.2004.03.030

[62] Casado A et al. Superoxide dismutase and catalase blood levels in patients with malignant diseases. Cancer Letters. 1995;**93**(2):187-192. DOI: 10.1016/0304-3835(95)03808-A

[63] Sousa RT et al. Oxidative stress in early stage bipolar disorder and the association with response to lithium. Journal of Psychiatric Research. 2014;**50**:36-41. DOI: 10.1016/j.jpsychires.2013.11.011

[64] Flohé L, Gunzler WA, Schock HH. Glutathione peroxidase: A selenoenzyme. FEBS Letters. 1973;**32**(1):132-134. DOI: 10.1016/0014-5793(73)80755-0

[65] Epp O, Ladenstein R, Wendel A. The refined structure of the selenoenzyme glutathione peroxidase at 0.2-nm resolution. European Journal of Biochemistry. 1983;**133**(1):51-69. DOI: 10.1111/j.1432-1033.1983.tb07429.x

[66] Lubos E, Loscalzo J, Handy DE. Glutathione peroxidase-1 in

health and disease: From molecular mechanisms to therapeutic opportunities. Antioxidants & Redox Signaling. 2011;**15**(7):1957-1997. DOI: 10.1089/ars.2010.3586

[67] Zimmermann R et al. Inhibition of lipid peroxidation in isolated inner membrane of rat liver mitochondria by superoxide dismutase. FEBS Letters. 1973;**29**(2):117-120. DOI: 10.1016/0014-5793(73)80539-3

[68] Gaetani GF et al. Predominant role of catalase in the disposal of hydrogen peroxide within human erythrocytes. Blood. 1996;**87**(4):1595-1599

[69] Cohen G, Hochstein P. Glutathione peroxidase: The primary agent for the elimination of hydrogen peroxide in erythrocytes. Biochemistry. 1963;**2**(6):1420-1428. DOI: 10.1021/bi00906a038

[70] Johnson RM et al. Hemoglobin autoxidation and regulation of endogenous H_2O_2 levels in erythrocytes. Free Radical Biology & Medicine. 2005;**39**(11):1407-1417. DOI: 10.1016/j.freeradbiomed.2005.07.002

[71] Flohé L et al. Glutathione peroxidase, V. The kinetic mechanism. Hoppe-Seyler's Zeitschrift für Physiologische Chemie. 1972;**353**(6):987-999

[72] Lee TH et al. Peroxiredoxin II is essential for sustaining life span of erythrocytes in mice. Blood. 2003;**101**(12):5033-5038. DOI: 10.1182/blood-2002-08-2548

[73] Low FM et al. Peroxiredoxin 2 functions as a noncatalytic scavenger of low-level hydrogen peroxide in the erythrocyte. Blood. 2007;**109**(6):2611-2617. DOI: 10.1182/blood-2006-09-048728

[74] Nagababu E et al. Role of peroxiredoxin-2 in protecting RBCs from hydrogen peroxide-induced oxidative stress. Free Radical Research. 2013;**47**(3):164-171. DOI: 10.3109/10715762.2012.756138

[75] Peskin AV et al. The high reactivity of peroxiredoxin 2 with H_2O_2 is not reflected in its reaction with other oxidants and thiol reagents. The Journal of Biological Chemistry. 2007;**282**(16):11885-11892. DOI: 10.1074/jbc.M700339200

[76] Ho YS et al. Mice lacking catalase develop normally but show differential sensitivity to oxidant tissue injury. The Journal of Biological Chemistry. 2004;**279**(31):32804-32812. DOI: 10.1074/jbc.M404800200

[77] Ogasawara Y et al. Structural and functional analysis of native peroxiredoxin 2 in human red blood cells. The International Journal of Biochemistry & Cell Biology. 2012;**44**(7):1072-1077. DOI: 10.1016/j.biocel.2012.04.008

[78] Jang HH et al. Two enzymes in one. Cell. 2004;**117**(5):625-635. DOI: 10.1016/j.cell.2004.05.002

[79] Han Y et al. Peroxiredoxin II is essential for preventing hemolytic anemia from oxidative stress through maintaining hemoglobin stability. Biochemical and Biophysical Research Communications. 2012;**426**(3):427-432. DOI: 10.1016/j.bbrc.2012.08.113

[80] Melo D, Ribeiro S, Santos-Silva A, Rocha S. Role of peroxiredoxin 2 in erythrocyte antioxidant defense: Peroxidase and chaperone. Free Radical Biological and Medicine. 2018;**120**(Suppl):S83. DOI: 10.1016/j.freeradbiomed.2018.04.274

[81] Moore RB et al. Reconstitution of $Ca(2^+)$-dependent K^+ transport in erythrocyte membrane vesicles requires a cytoplasmic protein. The

Journal of Biological Chemistry. 1991;**266**(28):18964-18968

[82] Brizuela M et al. Treatment of erythrocytes with the 2-cys peroxiredoxin inhibitor, Conoidin A, prevents the growth of Plasmodium falciparum and enhances parasite sensitivity to chloroquine. PLoS One. 2014;**9**(4):e92411. 1-8. DOI: 10.1371/journal.pone.0092411

[83] Memon A et al. Identification of differentially expressed proteins during human urinary bladder cancer progression. Cancer Detection and Prevention. 2005;**29**(3):249-255. DOI: 10.1016/j.cdp.2005.01.002

[84] Noh DY et al. Overexpression of peroxiredoxin in human breast cancer. Anticancer Research. 2001;**21**(3B):2085-2090

[85] Yoshida Y et al. Hydroxyoctadecadienoic acid and oxidatively modified peroxiredoxins in the blood of Alzheimer's disease patients and their potential as biomarkers. Neurobiology of Aging. 2009;**30**(2):174-185. DOI: 10.1016/j.neurobiolaging.2007.06.012

[86] Kwon HS et al. Hyperoxidized peroxiredoxins in peripheral blood mononuclear cells of asthma patients is associated with asthma severity. Life Sciences. 2012;**90**(13-14):502-508. DOI: 10.1016/j.lfs.2012.01.003

[87] Ogasawara Y et al. A simple high performance liquid chromatography method for quantitatively determining the reduced form of peroxiredoxin 2 and the mass spectrometric analysis of its oxidative status. Journal of Chromatography B. 2015;**997**:136-141. DOI: 10.1016/j.chromb.201506.007

[88] Mueller S, Riedel HD, Stremmel W. Direct evidence for catalase as the predominant H_2O_2 -removing enzyme in human erythrocytes. Blood. 1997;**90**(12):4973-4978

[89] Gaetani GF et al. Catalase and glutathione peroxidase are equally active in detoxification of hydrogen peroxide in human erythrocytes. Blood. 1989;**73**(1):334-339

[90] Johnson RM et al. Oxidation of glutathione peroxidase-deficient red cells by organic peroxides. Blood. 2002;**100**(4):1515-1516. DOI: 10.1182/blood-2002-04-1124

[91] Haruyama T et al. Negatively charged lipids are essential for functional and structural switch of human 2-Cys peroxiredoxin II. Journal of Molecular Biology. 2018;**430**(5):602-610. DOI: 10.1016/j.jmb.2017.12.020

[92] Matte A et al. Peroxiredoxin-2: A novel regulator of iron homeostasis in ineffective erythropoiesis. Antioxidants & Redox Signaling. 2018;**28**(1):1-14. DOI: 10.1089/ars.2017.7051

[93] Rinalducci S et al. Peroxiredoxin-2 as a candidate biomarker to test oxidative stress levels of stored red blood cells under blood bank conditions. Transfusion. 2011;**51**(7):1439-1449. DOI: 10.1111/j.1537-2995.2010.03032.x

[94] van Gestel RA et al. Quantitative erythrocyte membrane proteome analysis with blue-native/SDS PAGE. Journal of Proteomics. 2010;**73**(3):456-465. DOI: 10.1016/j.jprot.2009.08.010

[95] Allen DW et al. Increased membrane binding of erythrocyte catalase in hereditary spherocytosis and in metabolically stressed normal cells. Blood. 1977;**49**(1):113-123

[96] Bayer SB et al. Interactions between peroxiredoxin 2, hemichrome and the erythrocyte membrane. Free Radical Research. 2016;**50**(12):1329-1339. DOI: 10.1080/10715762.2016.1241995

[97] D'Alessandro A et al. Time-course investigation of SAGM-stored leukocyte-filtered red bood cell concentrates: From metabolism to proteomics. Haematologica. 2012;**97**(1):107-115. DOI: 10.3324/haematol.2011.051789

[98] Matte A et al. Membrane association of peroxiredoxin-2 in red cells is mediated by the N-terminal cytoplasmic domain of band 3. Free Radical Biology & Medicine. 2013;**55**:27-35. DOI: 10.1016/j.freeradbiomed.2012.10.543

[99] Matte A et al. Peroxiredoxin-2 expression is increased in beta-thalassemic mouse red cells but is displaced from the membrane as a marker of oxidative stress. Free Radical Biology & Medicine. 2010;**49**(3):457-466. DOI: 10.1016/j.freeradbiomed.2010.05.003

Chapter 7

Effects of Therapeutic and Toxic Agents on Erythrocytes of Different Species of Animals

Saganuwan Alhaji Saganuwan

Abstract

A preponderance of therapeutic and toxic agents that affect erythrocytes is being used in preclinical and clinical settings. Such agents are responsible for wrong diagnosis of a myriad of diseases and poor prognosis of some therapeutic interventions. In view of this, literature search was carried out with a view to investigate morphometry of erythrocytes in various diseased conditions and species of animals. Findings have shown that erythrocyte size, area, and volume vary in different species of animals under different diseased conditions. Environmental factors, toxicants, toxins, therapeutics, and management system, among others, can cause erythrocyte deformation, leading to anemia. Erythrocyte-related diseases include but not limited to sickle cell anemia, malaria, cancer, psychiatric illness, and chronic inflammation. Hence the principal source of our survival is erythrocyte, because it transports oxygen needed for metabolism of cell nutrients.

Keywords: drug, toxin, toxicant, size, shape, erythrocyte, blood disease, treatment, allometry

1. Introduction

Blood is a connective tissue comprising hematocrit (45%), white blood cells, platelets, red blood cells, and plasma (55%) which is a mixture of protein, water, lipids, amino acids, hormone, carbohydrates, vitamins, and cellular wastes [1]. About 8% of body weight is blood [2, 3], 18% protein and water substances, 15% fat, 7% mineral, and 60% water [4]. Increased surface area of erythrocytes is an adaptation for transportation of oxygen bound to hemoglobin [5]. But destruction of RBCs can lead to anemia based on cause and morphology of erythrocytes. Anemia could be hereditary [6], sickle cell anemia, Mediterranean anemia (thalassemia), glucose-6-phosphate dehydrogenase (6GPD) anemia, aplastic anemia, hemolytic disease of newborn, and acquired hemolytic anemia [7]. Fresh frozen plasma and plasma protein can serve as expander and supply clotting for patients with clotting factor-deficient diseases [8]. Blood can be collected from mice and rat tail, lateral saphenous vein, lateral tail vein, retro-orbital sinus, and heart. Only 1% of blood should be collected at a time [9]. Plasma expanders exert oncotic pressure during infusion and are retained in the vascular compartment [10]. Bed rest of 100–200 days decreased plasma volume by 30% [11]. Blood count consists of erythrocytes, hematocrit, hemoglobin, leucocytes, and differential leucocyte counts. The normal range of erythrocytes (4.2–6.2 × 10^{12}/L), hemoglobin (100 g/100 mL), and hematocrit (38–54%) of the total blood volume are the standards for human species [12]. Variation in species, age, environmental factors, management system, and pathological conditions could affect the size, shape, area, and volume of erythrocytes.

2. Methodology

Extensive literature search was carried out to identify differences between normal and abnormal erythrocytes of various species of animals including the ones in the wild. Information on beneficial and toxic effects of drugs, chemical toxicants, toxins, plant extracts, chemicals, and diseased conditions were searched on erythrocyte shape, size, and volume for various species of animals including human. Some developed formulas were modified for determination of anemic, polycythemic, hydrated, and dehydrated erythrocytes. Physiological and pathological features of the erythrocytes were also highlighted. Preclinical and clinical values of the changes in erythrocytes in relation to blood diseases caused by various agents were critically analyzed. Effects of toxic and therapeutic agents on metabolic, cancer, infectious, inheritable, and noninheritable diseases of erythrocytes, such as sickle cell anemia, malaria, and hereditary spherocytosis, among others, were elucidated.

3. Results

The values of erythrocytes, packed cell volume plasma volume, hemoglobin concentration, body weight, and salient features of erythrocytes are presented in **Table 1**, **Figures 1–23** [26, 27].

3.1 Morphometry of erythrocytes

Erythrocytes have larger (a) and minor (b) axes, volume (v), and surface area. The measurement is in micrometer (μm):

$$a = \frac{1}{2}; b = \frac{1}{2}.$$

$$\text{Surface area} = 2a^2\left(1 + \frac{c}{ac}\text{sine}^{-1}e\right); \text{where } e^{-1} = 1\frac{-a^2}{c^2} \quad (1)$$

$$\text{Volume} = {}^4\!/_3\, a^2 \times b \quad (2)$$

Hematological variances can occur between animals of different species and the same species. Erythrocytes of *Piaractus mesopotamicus* (2.57 ± 0.5 × $10^6/\mu l$) was higher than that of *Brycon orbignyanus* (2.56 ± 0.5 × $10^6/\mu l$), *Oreochromis niloticus* (1.70 ± 0.4 × $10^6/\mu l$), and *Rhamdia quelen* (2.11 ± 0.6 × $10^6/\mu l$), respectively. Larger axes of *R. quelen* (12.1 ± 0.3 μm), *O. niloticus* (13.2 ± 0.6 μm), *B. orbignyanus* (14.4 ± 0.3 μm), and *P. mesopotamicus* (15.0 ± 0.4 μm), as compared to their minor axes, 9.3 ± 0.3, 9.3 ± 0.4, 8.7 ± 0.2, and 9.8 ± 0.2 μm, respectively, as well as the surface area and volume of *R. quelen* (317.0 ± 36.4 μm^2; 545.2 ± 95.0 μm^3), *O. niloticus* (343.1 ± 43.4 μm^2; 612.6 ± 119.4 μm^3), *B. orbignyanus* (337.3 ± 30.771 μm^2; 585.4 ± 84.0 μm^3), and *P. mesopotamicus* (400.6 ± 36.5 μm^2; 765.8 ± 108.7 μm^3), respectively, show that erythrocyte shape, area, and volume vary even in the same species of animals [28].

Breed	English name	Scientific name	Weight (kg)	Erythrocytes ($\times 10^6/\mu l$)	Hematocrit	Hemoglobin concentration (g/dl)	Plasma volume (ml)	Total blood volume (ml)	Comment(s)	References
Canis	Dog	*Canis familiaris*	7.19	6.12 ± 0.25	36.75 ± 1.49	12.25 ± 0.49	363.8	575.2	High blood volume	[13]
Mus	Mouse	*Mus musculus*	0.025	9.60 ± 1.02	36.00 ± 2.58	11.90 ± 0.86	1.28	2.0	High plasma volume	[14]
Meleagris	Turkey	*Meleagris gallopavo*	2.0	1.99–2.26	33.2 ± 3.56	11.07±1.19	106.9	160	High plasma volume	[15]
Mus	Mouse	*Mus musculus*	0.021	1.09 ± 0.04	41.00 ± 2.08	13.67±0.69	1.0	1.7	High hematocrit	[16]
Rattus	Rat	*Rattus norvegicus*	0.16	7.21±0.14	38.17±0.87	13.83±0.06	7.9	12.8	High erythrocytes	[17]
Caprine	Goat	*Capra hircus*	13	11.5±0.4	29.4±0.8	9.8±0.3	734.2	1040	Higher erythrocytes	[18]
Labeo	Fish	*Labeo rohita*	1.48	1.3±0.03	24.30±3.30	8.1±1.10	89.6	118.4	Lower hematocrit	[19]
Struthio	Ostrich	*Struthio camelus*	111	151.58±0.30	36.47±3.78	11.37±0.70	5641.7	8880	Very high erythrocytes	[20]
Streptopelia	Laughing dove	*Streptopelia senegalensis*	0.1	3.76±0.01	42.60±0.86	14.04±0.25	4.6	8.0	Higher hematocrit	[21]
Naja	Indian cobra	*Naja naja*	9.3	0.58±0.04	30.11±1.93	7.6±0.75	520	744	Lower hemoglobin	[22]
Bos	Cow	*Bos indicus*	450	6.7 ± 0.65	28.50±2.05	7.55±3.5	25,740	36,000	Lower hematocrit	[23]
Homo	Child	*Homo sapiens*	23.25	0.36–0.28	24.33–19.09	7.81–4.59	1407.5-1505	1860	Lower parameters	[24]
Homo	Man	*Homo sapiens*	70	4.5–5.9	39–49	13.6–17.2	2856.1–3416.1	5600	Lower plasma volume	[25]
Homo	Woman	*Homo sapiens*	70	3.5–5.0	33–43	12.0–15.0	3192.2–3752.1	5600	Higher plasma volume	[25]

Key: Hemoglobin = 1/3 of hematocrit.

Table 1.
Erythrocytes, packed cell volume, and hemoglobin concentration in various species of animals.

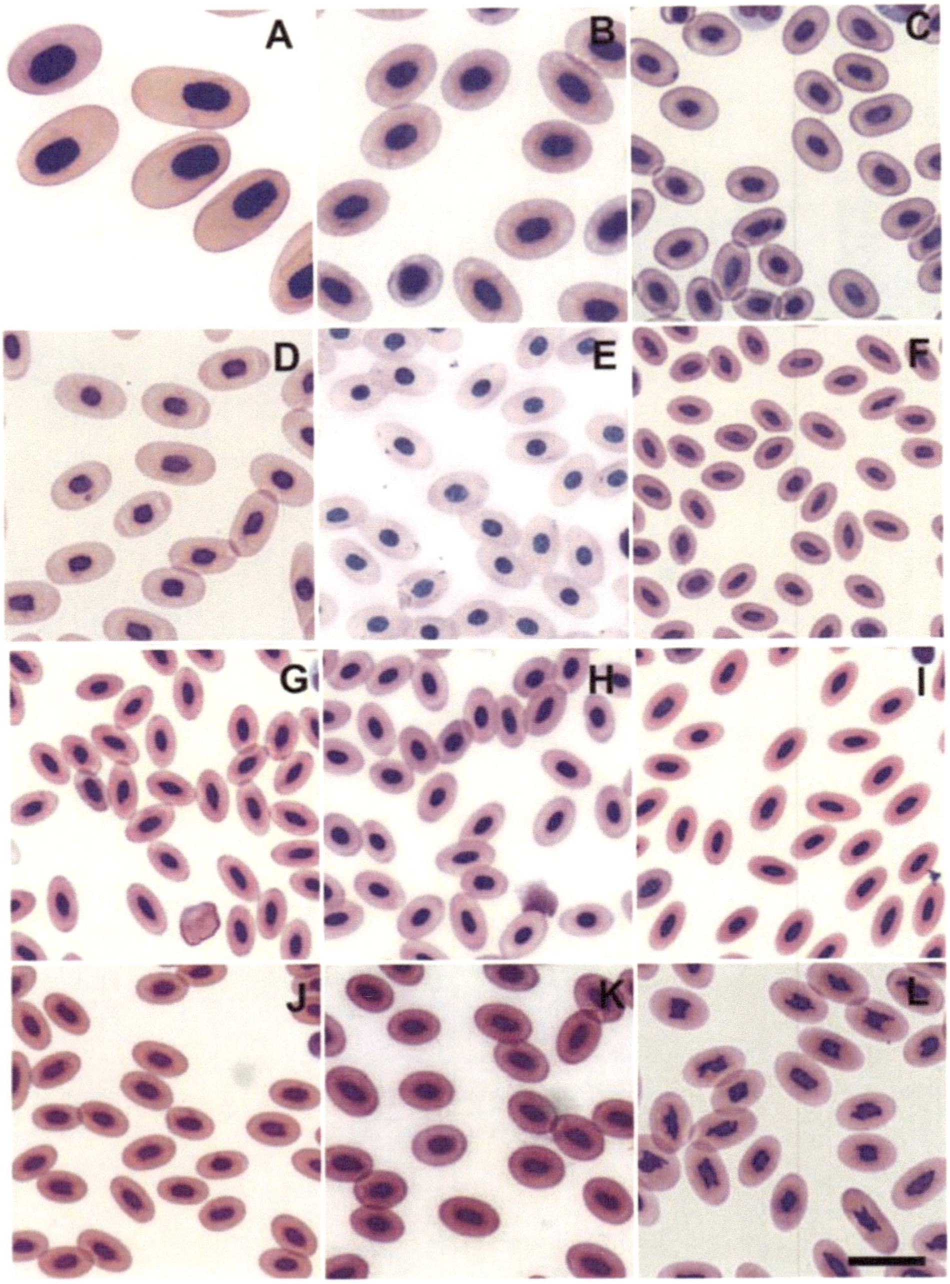

Figure 1.
Photomicrographs of erythrocytes of some amphibian and reptile species. (A) O. vittatus, (B) P. caralitanus, (C) P. caucasicus, (D) E. orbicularis, (E) T. graeca, (F) O. elegans, (G) M. brevirostris, (H) A. danfordi, (I) L. trilineata, (J) L. macrorhynchus, (K) H. ravergieri, (L) M. xanthina.

4. Discussion

4.1 Erythrocytes in various species of animals

Erythrocytes in various species of animals vary both in quality and quantity. For example, lactating Holstein breed of cow had hematocrit of 28.50 ± 2.05% and hemoglobin of 7.55 ± 3.5 g/dl on the first lactation and hematocrit (30.02 ± 2.05%)

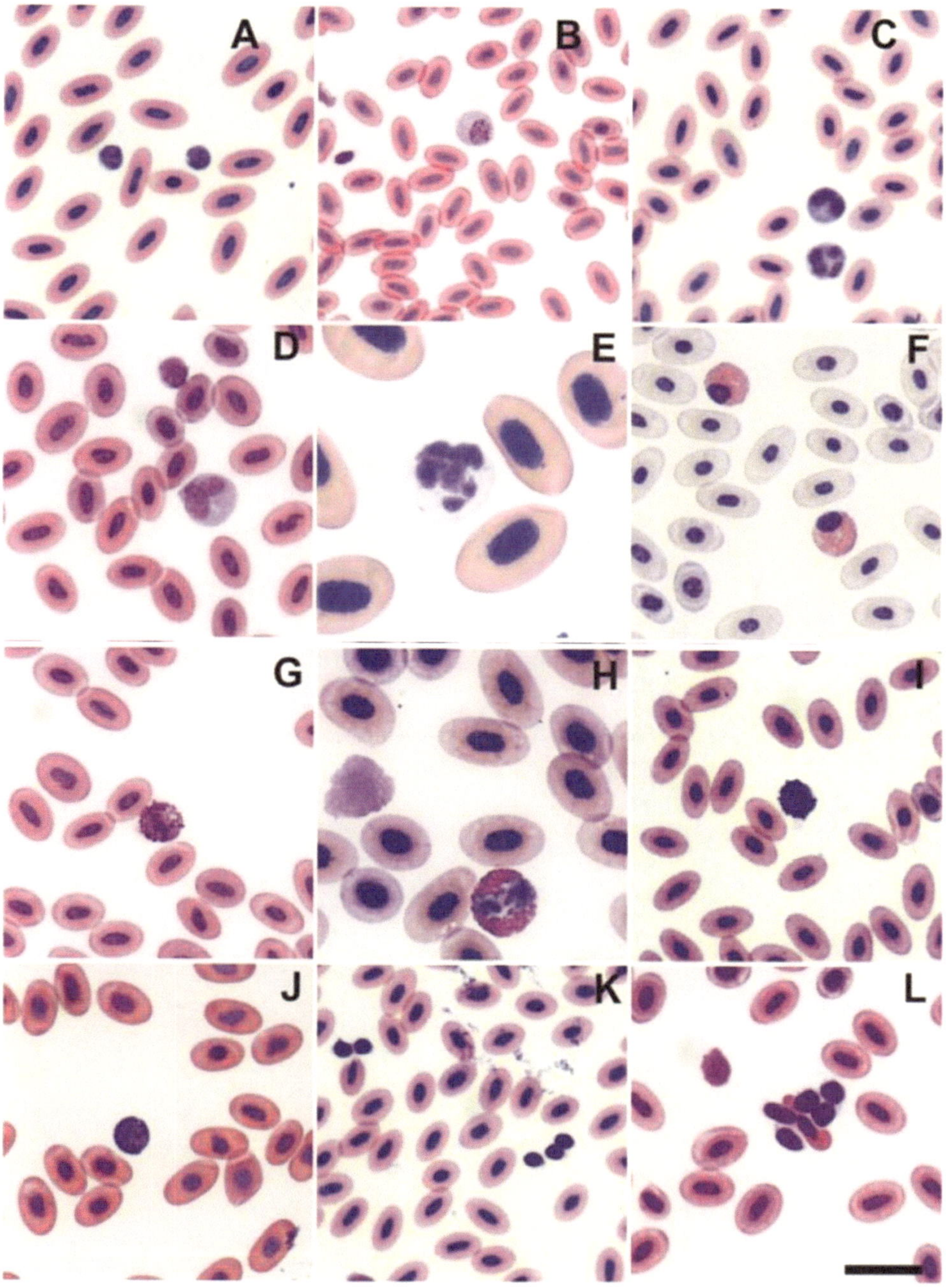

Figure 2.
Photomicrographs of leukocytes and thrombocytes in some amphibian and reptile species. (A) small lymphocyte (L. trilineata), (B) large lymphocyte (Z. hohenackeri), (C) monocyte and heterophil (O. elegans), (D) monocyte (P. najadum), (E) heterophil (N. strauchi), (F) heterophil (T. hermanni), (G) eosinophil (P. najadum), (H) eosinophil (P. caralitanus), (I) basophil (A. cappadocica), (J) basophil (S. diadema), (K) a group of thrombocytes (O. elegans), (L) a group of thrombocytes (P. najadum).

and hemoglobin (12.5 ± 2.1 g/dl) on the sixth lactation, respectively. Hence frequency of lactations changes erythrocytes in dairy cow. Albumin (2.92 ± 0.17 g/dl) on the first lactation increased to 3.69 ± 0.08 g/dl on the sixth lactation, respectively [23]. Hence increased erythrocytes may connote increased albumin. Ostrich (*Struthio camelus*) could weigh between 70 and 150 kg. The erythrocytes (151.58 ± 0.30 × 10^6/mm^3), hemoglobin (11.37 ± 0.70 g/dl), and hematocrit (36.47 ± 3.78%)

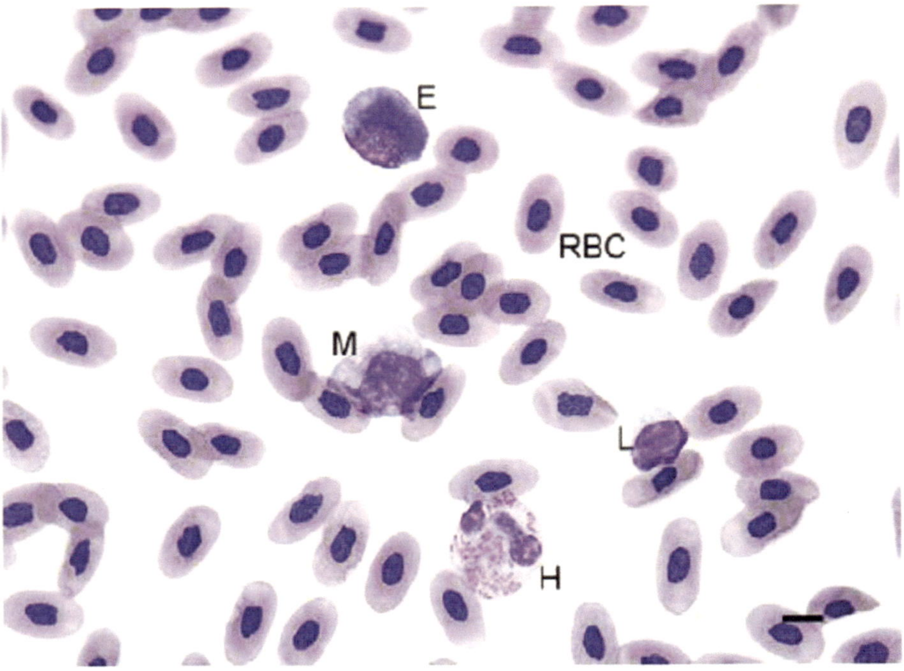

Figure 3.
Peripheral blood from a clinically healthy green iguana (Iguana iguana). E, green eosinophil; H, bilobed heterophil; L, lymphocyte; M, monocyte; RBC.

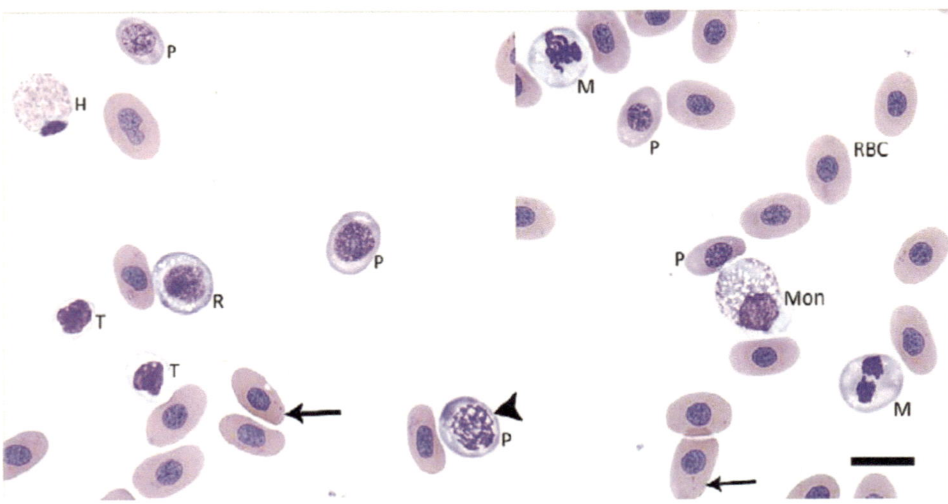

Figure 4.
Peripheral blood from a green sea turtle (Chelonia mydas) with anemia (PCV 5–12%) and evidence of erythroid regeneration. Mature erythrocytes (RBC) with mild basophilic stippling (arrows). Polychromatophil undergoing mitosis (arrowhead). H, heterophil; M, mitotic figures in erythroid cell line; Mon, reactive monocyte; P, polychromatophils; R, rubriblast; T, thrombocytes.

of ostrich chick were higher than erythrocytes ($131.83 \pm 0.19 \times 10^6/mm^3$), hemoglobin ($12.01 \pm 1.51$ g/dl), and hematocrit ($40.15 \pm 2.44\%$) of grower ostrich. Total protein was higher (4.32 ± 0.29 g/dl) in ostrich chick than that of young ostrich (3.63 ± 0.54 g/dl), respectively [20], signifying that total protein may be correlated with erythrocytes. Hematocrit of Kano brown buck ($55.8 \pm 1.12\%$) is higher than that of Kano brown doe ($31.0 \pm 0.73\%$), Borno white buck ($34.00 \pm 1.2\%$), Kano brown doe ($8.80 \pm 0.44\%$), Sokoto red doe ($8.2 \pm 0.34\%$), and Sokoto red buck

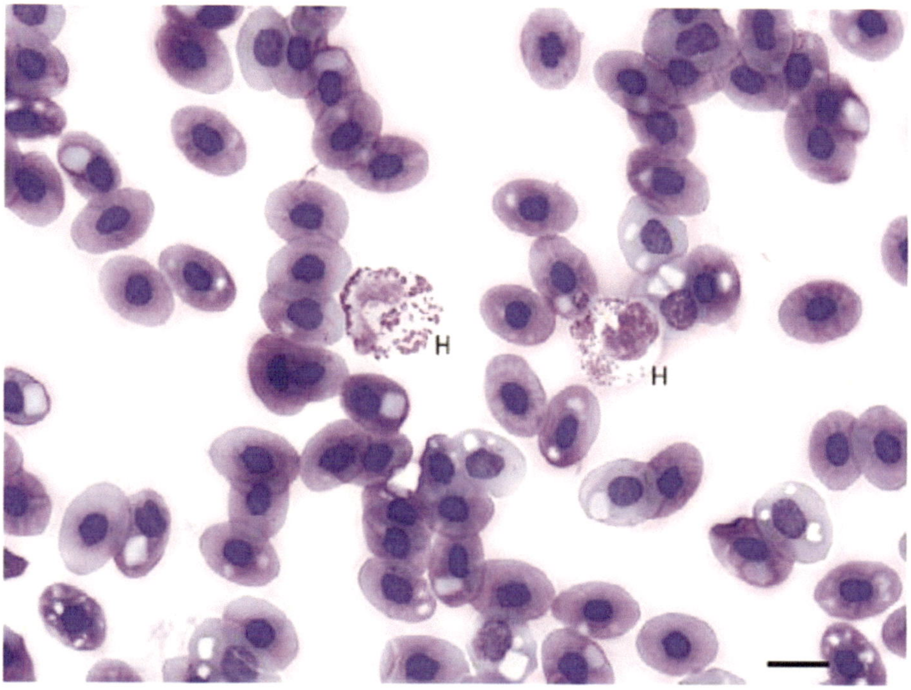

Figure 5.
Peripheral blood from a clinically healthy green iguana (Iguana iguana). Erythrocytes contain variably sized, pale rectangular to square cytoplasmic inclusions of unknown origin. H, bilobed heterophils.

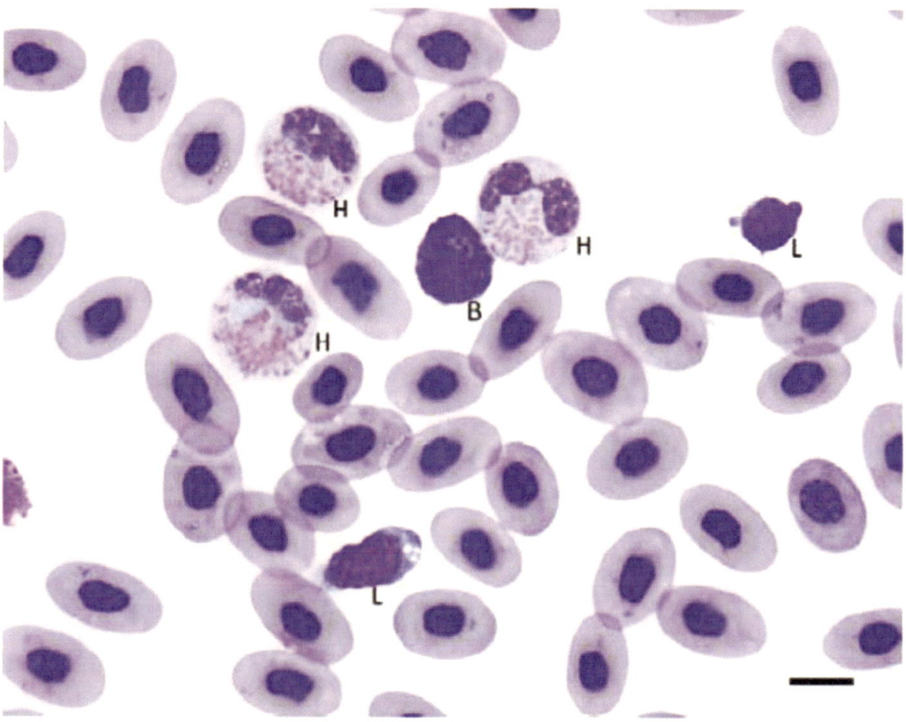

Figure 6.
Peripheral blood from a Chinese dragon (Physignathus cocincinus) with multiple subcutaneous abscesses and heterophilia. Heterophils (H) are mildly toxic (degranulation and cytoplasmic basophilia). Erythrocytes are mature and contain small, pale basophilic inclusions consistent with degenerate organelles. B, basophil; L, small lymphocytes.

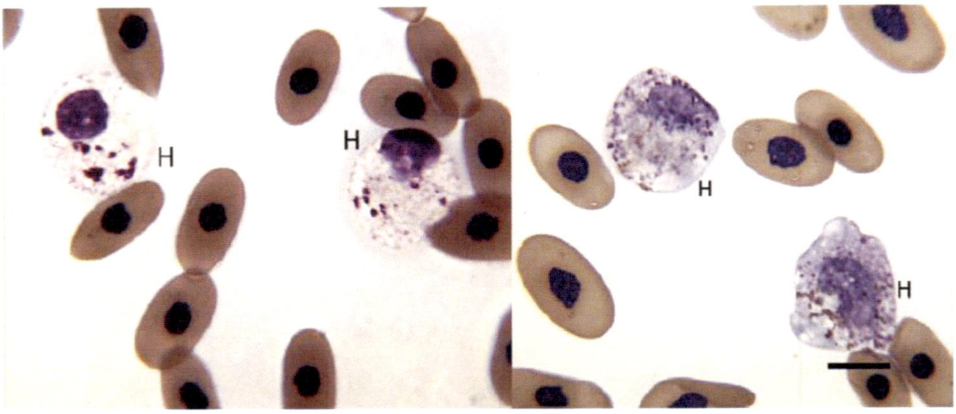

Figure 7.
Peripheral blood from (left) an American crocodile (Crocodylus acutus) and (right) a spectacled caiman (Caiman crocodilus). Heterophils (H) are severely toxic, with degranulation, indistinct cytoplasmic vacuolation, and abnormal granules. The caiman heterophils also have increased cytoplasmic basophilia and immature nuclei.

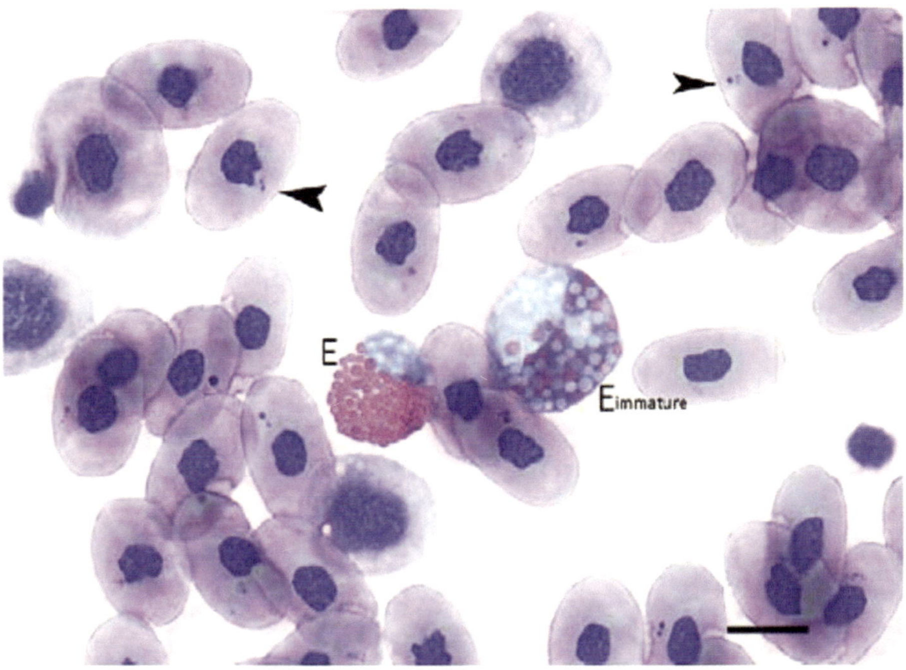

Figure 8.
Peripheral blood from a clinically healthy flowerback box turtle (Cuora galbinifrons). A mature eosinophil (E) and an immature eosinophil (Eimmature). A few of the mature erythrocytes contain small, basophilic inclusions consistent with degenerate organelles (arrowheads). P, polychromatophils.

(8.00 ± 0.29%), respectively. Erythrocytes of Sokoto red doe kid (1.96 ± 0.5 × 10^6/mm^3) are lower than that of buck kid (2.56 ± 6.11 × 10^6/mm^3), Kano brown buck kid (3.4 ± 0.01 × 10^6/ mm^3), and Kano brown doe kid (4.9 ± 6.11 × 10^6/mm^3), respectively. But total protein of Borno white buck (47 ± 1.2 g/dl) is lower than that of Sokoto red buck (69.0 ± 1.33 g/dl), whereas albumin of Borno white doe (26.00 ± 1.1 g/dl) is lower than that of Sokoto red doe (29.0 ± 0.06 g/dl), respectively [29]. Factors affecting erythrocyte management system such as intensive, semi-intensive, and extensive systems of grazing could change erythrocytes. Cattle under intensive care had erythrocytes at the beginning of grazing (6.62 × 10^6/mm^3)

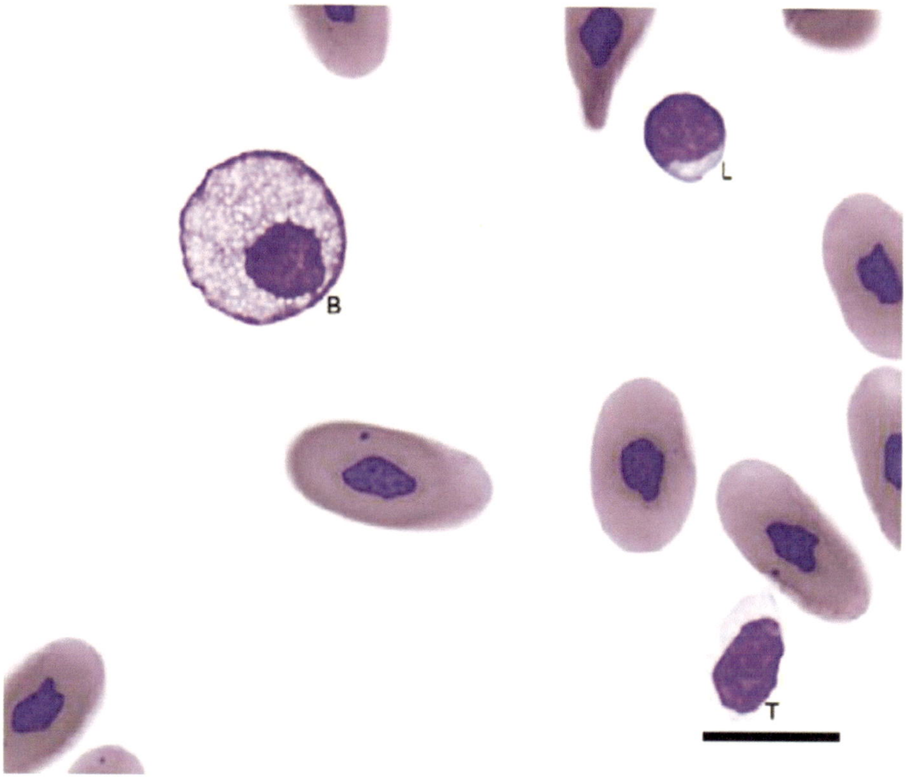

Figure 9.
Peripheral blood from a clinically healthy American alligator (Alligator mississippiensis). B, degranulated basophil; L, small lymphocyte; T, thrombocyte.

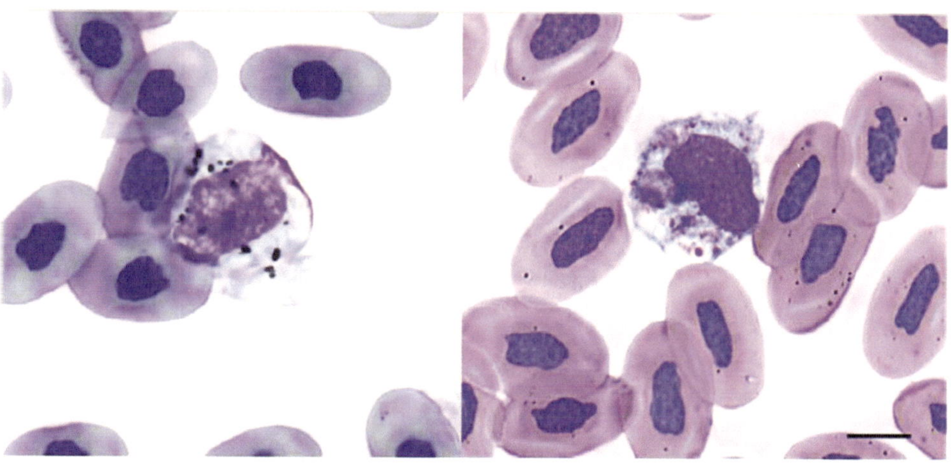

Figure 10.
Macrophages in peripheral blood. (Left) Melanomacrophage in a clinically healthy loggerhead sea turtle (Caretta caretta). (Right) Macrophage with intracytoplasmic nucleoproteinaceous debris in a common boa constrictor (Boa constrictor imperator). Macrophages are occasionally observed in the blood of clinically normal reptiles.

as compared to the end of grazing ($6.29 \times 10^6/mm^3$). However, those under extensive care had an erythrocyte increase of $6.69 \times 10^6/mm^3$ at the beginning of grazing and $7.26 \times 10^6/mm^3$ after grazing. But cattle that grazed on pasture in group had erythrocytes of $6.93 \times 10^6/mm^3$ at the beginning in comparison with $7.23 \times 10^6/mm^3$

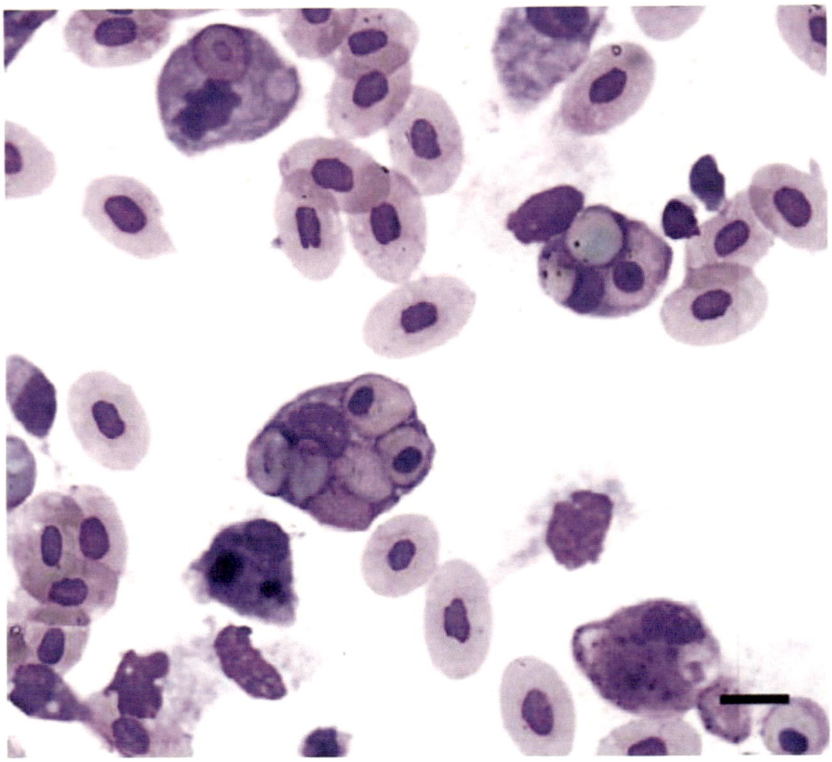

Figure 11.
Peripheral blood from an emerald tree boa (Corallus caninus) with positive blood culture for Corynebacterium sp. Several monocytes (macrophages) contain phagocytized erythrocytes and greenish black hemosiderin pigment. The cell in the upper left appears mitotic.

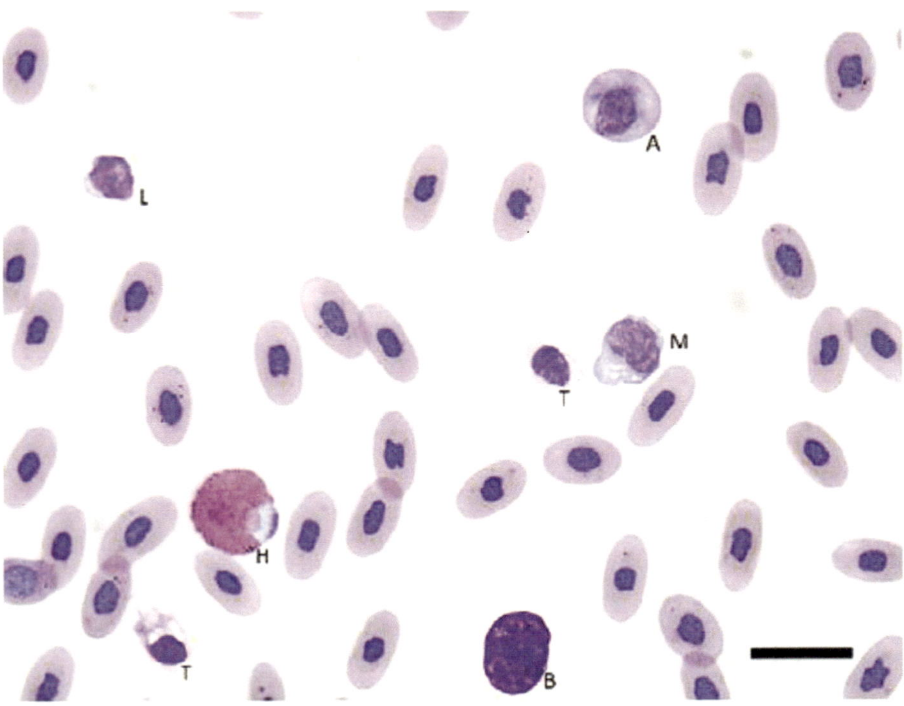

Figure 12.
Peripheral blood from a blood python (Python brongersmai) with chronic constipation. A, azurophil; B, basophil; H, heterophil; L, small lymphocyte; M, mildly vacuolated monocyte; T, thrombocytes, and mature erythrocytes.

DOI: http://dx.doi.org/10.5772/intechopen.85865

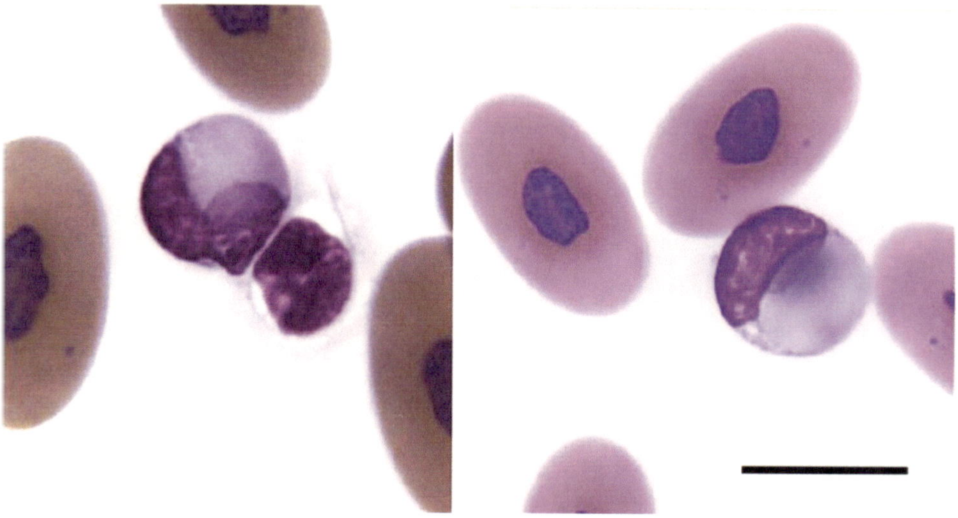

Figure 13.
Peripheral blood from (left) a rainbow boa (Epicrates cenchria cenchria) and (right) a common boa constrictor (Boa constrictor imperator) with inclusion body disease. Lymphocytes contain homogenous basophilic inclusions that displace the nucleus. A partially lysed thrombocyte is also seen in the image on the left.

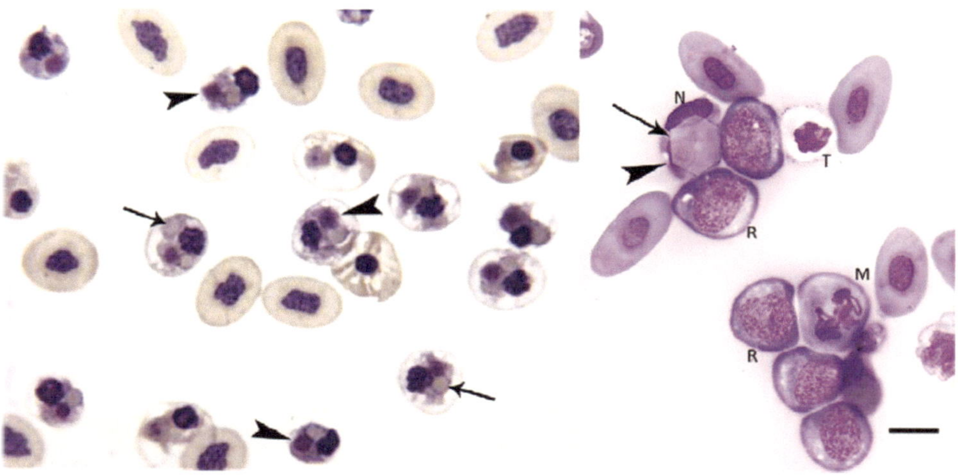

Figure 14.
Peripheral blood from a peninsula ribbon snake (Thamnophis sauritus sackenii) (left) and terciopelo (Bothrops asper) (right) with SEV infections. The erythrocytes contain crystalline inclusions (arrows) and granular eosinophilic viral inclusions (arrowheads) characteristic of SEV. Nucleus (N) of an erythroid precursor that contains a viral inclusion. M, mitotic figure; R, rubricyte; T, thrombocyte.

after grazing. Total protein was significantly higher in all the groups before grazing as compared to after grazing [30]. Erythrocytes of Nigerian laughing dove (*Streptopelia senegalensis*) after 4 weeks and 8 weeks in captivity are 3.76 ± 0.01 and 3.01 ± 0.11 $\times 10^6/\mu l$, respectively. The PCV after 4 weeks (42.60 ± 0.86%) was higher than after 8 weeks (34.60 ± 1.47%), respectively. Hemoglobin was significantly higher after 4 weeks (14.04 ± 0.25 g/dl) than 11.26 ± 0.48 g/dl after 8 weeks. But total protein and albumin were slightly lower after 4 weeks than after 8 weeks, suggesting that captivity could lead to decreased erythrocyte count [21]. Erythrocytes of West African dwarf goats are 11.5 ± 0.4 × $10^6/mm^3$, hematocrit is 29.4 ±0.8%, and hemoglobin is 9.8 ± 0.3 g/dl, respectively, whereas total protein and albumin are 7.1 ± 01 g/dl and 2.4 ± 0.7 g/dl, respectively [18]. Increase in erythrocytes, hemoglobin, and lactate in *Mugil cephalus* (fish) in comparison with other species of fish

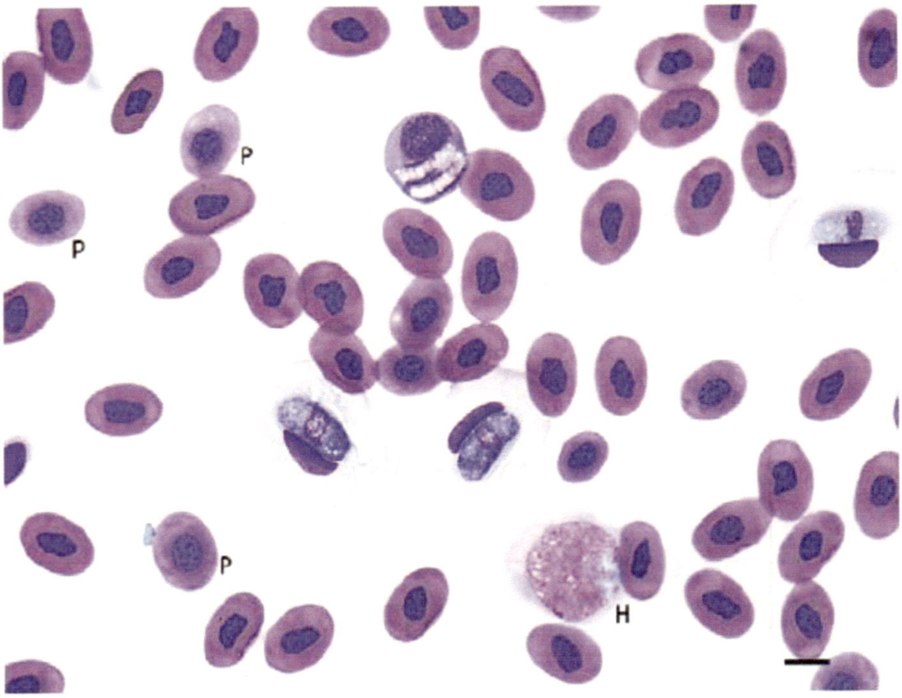

Figure 15.
Peripheral blood from an eastern indigo snake (Drymarchon corais couperi) with Hepatozoon sp. infection. Gametocytes can be seen in three highly swollen erythrocytes and one rubricyte. H, heterophil; P, polychromatophils.

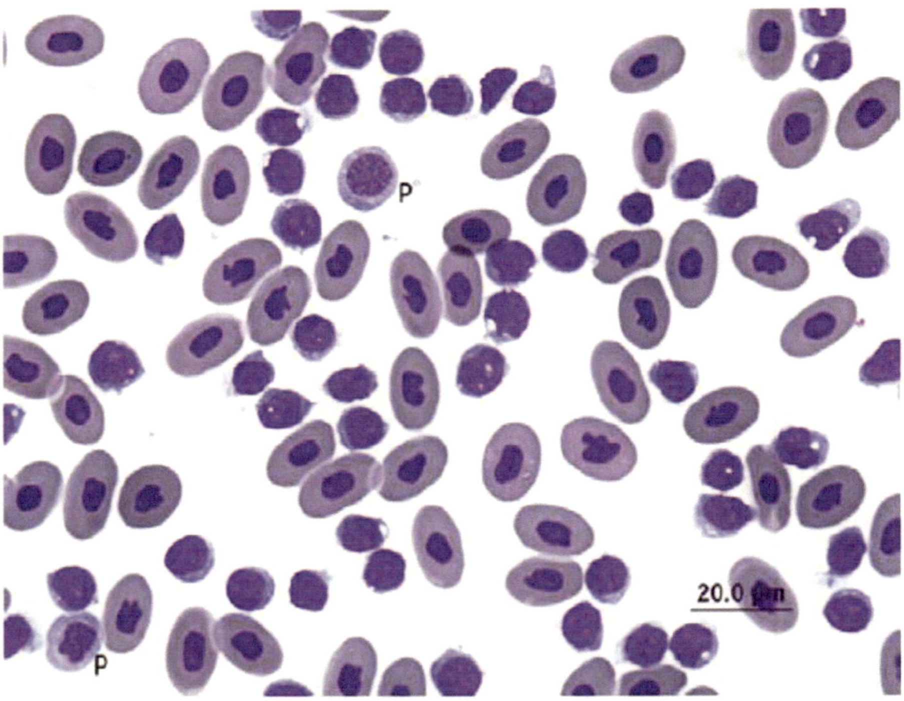

Figure 16.
Peripheral blood from an Asian cobra (Naja naja kaouthia) with marked leukocytosis (388,000/ml) diagnosed as a chronic lymphocytic leukemia. Neoplastic lymphocytes (L), polychromatophils (P). Lymphocytes were identified as T cell in origin by using immunocytochemistry.

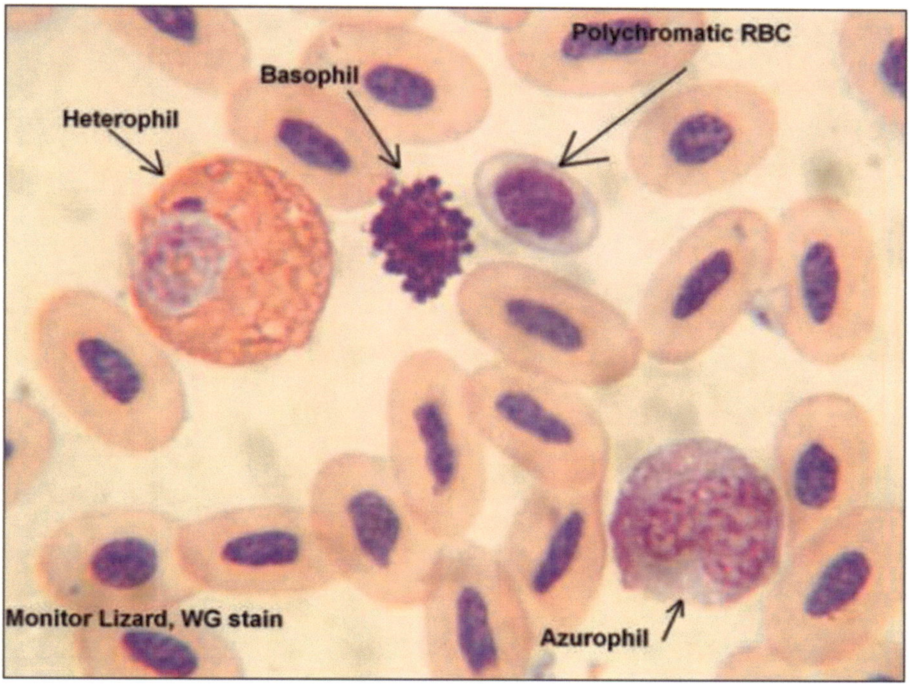

Figure 17.
Blood smear from a monitor lizard (Varanus sp.). Note the size, shape, and color of the polychromatic erythrocyte.

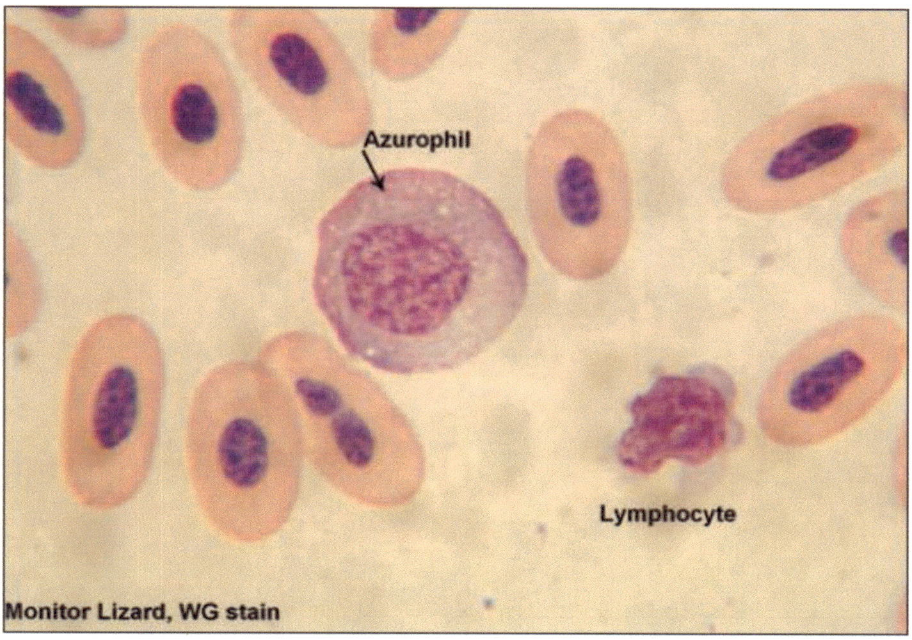

Figure 18.
Blood smear from a monitor lizard (Varanus sp.). Azurophils (center) have a round to oval nucleus and blue cytoplasm and contain very fine azurophilic granules. Lymphocytes are round to irregularly shaped, have an eccentric nucleus with dense chromatin, and have a large nuclear: cytoplasmic ratio.

such as *Gobius niger*, *Sparus aurata*, and *Dicentrarchus labrax* could be attributed to their feeding behavior, adaptation to the environment, and lifestyle [31]. Erythrocyte count of Balami ewe ($9.66 \pm 0.12 \times 10^6/mm^3$) is higher than that of

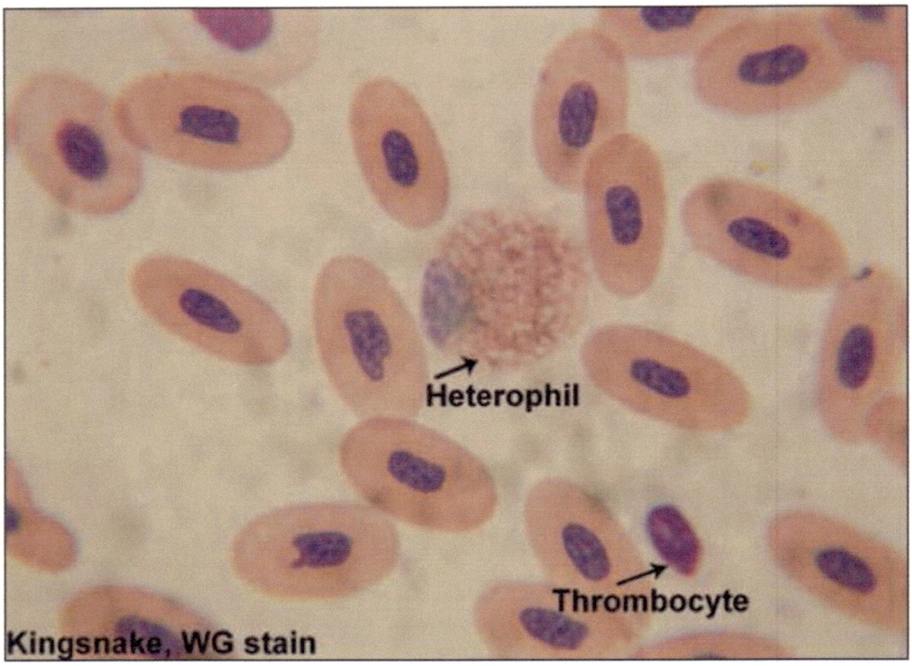

Figure 19.
Blood smear from a kingsnake (Lampropeltis sp.). Thrombocytes are often in clusters. The heterophil in the center is densely packed with granules, making the granular shapes almost indistinguishable.

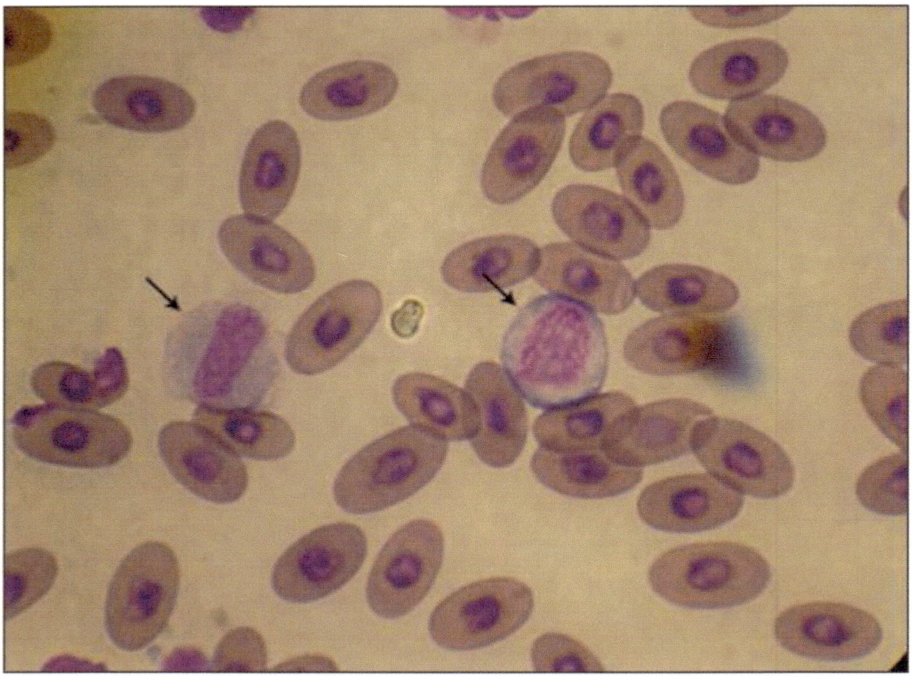

Figure 20.
Blood smear showing monocytes (arrows) from a green iguana (Iguana iguana).

Yankasa ewe ($9.31 \pm 0.78 \times 10^6/mm^3$), Ouda ewe ($9.25 \pm 0.02 \times 10^6/mm^3$), Yankasa ram ($7.80 \pm 0.62 \times 10^6/mm^3$), Balami ram ($7.21 \pm 0.42 \times 10^6/mm^3$), and Ouda ram ($6.49 \pm 0.01 \times 10^6/mm^3$), respectively. Ouda ram has the highest PCV value of 64 ± 2.14%, whereas Yankasa ram has the least PCV value of 28.90 ± 0.02%

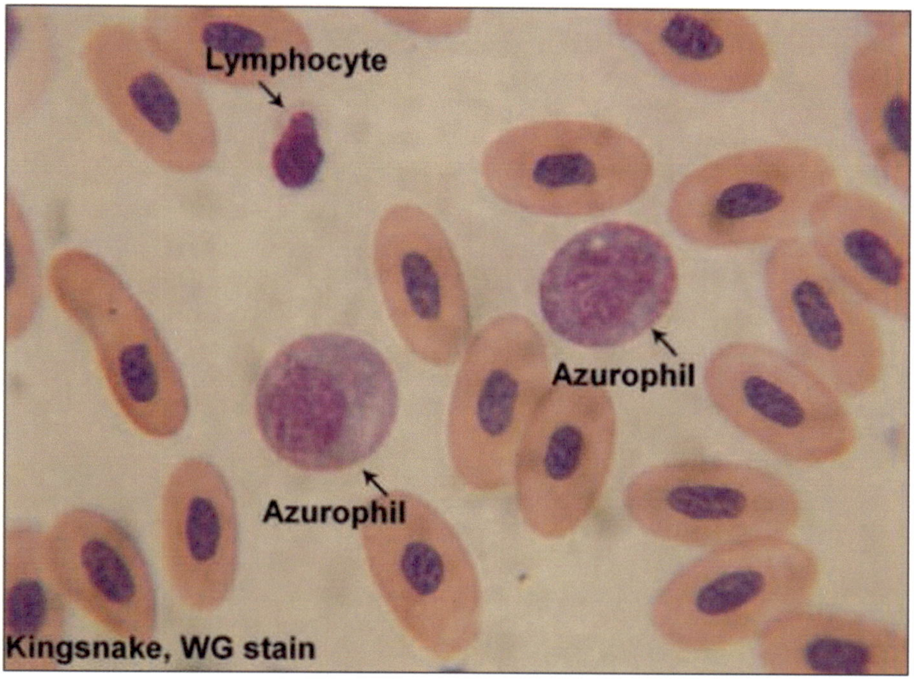

Figure 21.
Blood smear from a kingsnake (Lampropeltis sp.) showing two azurophils and a lymphocyte.

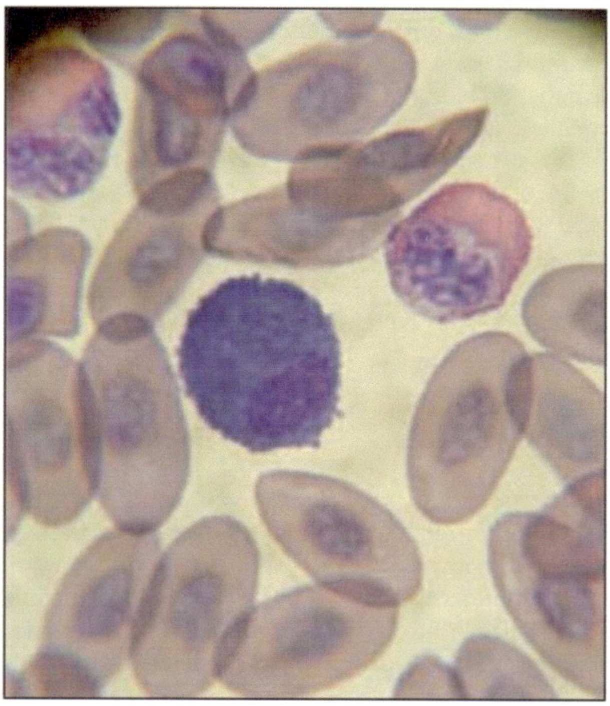

Figure 22.
Blood smear from a green iguana (Iguana iguana). In some species of reptiles, eosinophils contain blue granules (center). Two heterophils are also present.

[32]. Reference value for erythrocytes in cow (5–10 × $10^6/mm^3$) and PCV for sheep (24–45%), cow (24–48%), rabbit (30–50%), guinea pig (37–48%), and swine (32–50%), respectively, show that swine has the highest PCV value in this group of

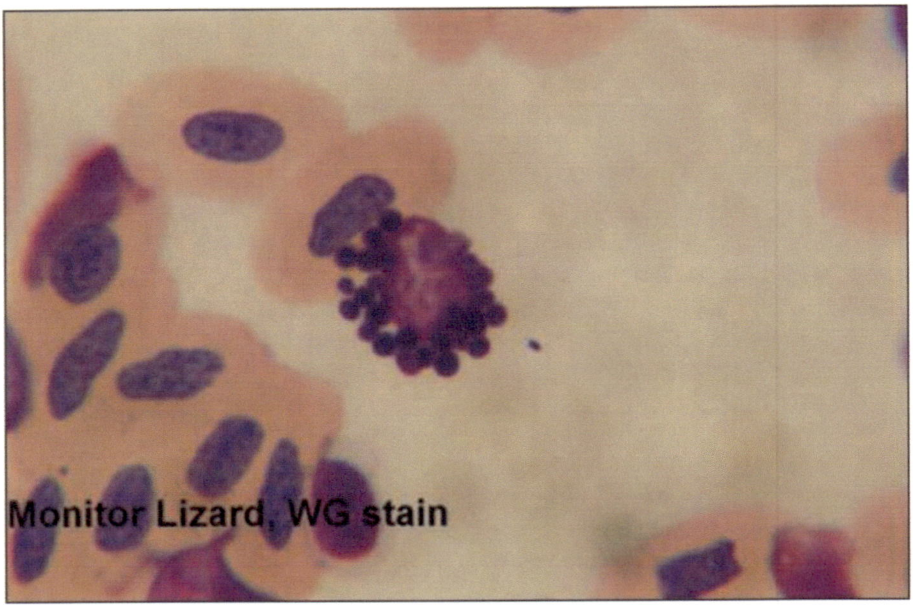

Figure 23.
Blood smear from a monitor lizard (Varanus sp.). Slight distortion of the basophil (center) reveals the nucleus and granules.

animals. But reference value of hemoglobin concentration for swine (10–16 g/dl), sheep (8–16 g/dl), cow (15–18 g/dl), rabbit (10–15 g/dl), and guinea pig (11–15 g/dl), respectively, indicates that cow has the highest hemoglobin concentration, perhaps resulting from hemolysis. Toxicants, environmental factors, genetics, age, sex, breed, and management system could affect erythrocytes of farm animals [33]. An image-based error (3%) for counting of RBCs has been reported for *Leopardus pardalis*, *Cebus apella*, and *Nasua nasua*. However the RBC values for *Canis familiaris* (5.50–8.50 $\times$ 10^6/mm^3), *Equus caballus* (6.10–11.0 $\times$ 10^6/mm^3), *Leopardus pardalis* (4.07–6.16 $\times$ 10^6/mm^3), *Cebus apella* (3.49–5.48 $\times$ 10^6/mm^3), and *Nasua nasua* (3.88–5.35 $\times$ 10^6/mm^3) with the species showing RBC interval of 3.47–11.0 $\times$ 10^6/μl) [34], respectively, show that erythrocyte volume varies from species to species of animals.

4.2 Diseases of erythrocytes

But changes in erythrocyte shape, area, and volume may be caused by malaria, sickle cell disease, and other related erythrocytes diseases. Malaria parasites of clinical and laboratory importance include *P. falciparum*, *P. vivax*, *P. malariae*, *P. ovale*, and *P. knowlesi* in human and could be treated using orthodox and traditional medicine [35]. The gorilla, chimpanzee, orangutan, gibbon, and monkey also contract various species of malaria. *Aotus trivirgatus* (species of monkey) are experimental models for human *P. vivax* and *P. falciparum*. *P. berghei* discovered in *Grammomys sudaster* is a model of experiment for mammalian malaria. Mice and young rats could also be used as models for *P. berghei* which is very fatal, causing death in 1–3 weeks when less than 10^7 *P. berghei* was inoculated. *P. relictum*, *P. gallinaceum*, *P. cathemerium*, and *P. lophurae* are also used as models of experiment. *P. durae* and *P. juxtanucleare* caused 96% mortality in turkey [36] indicating that malaria could be a source of low erythrocyte count in all the species mentioned above. Consistent acridine orange staining of thin blood film for malaria parasites and rapid staining tests produce superior results in comparison to Giemsa method [37].

Sickle cell disease (SCD) is characterized by dense dehydrated red blood cells (DRBCs) that undergo polymerization and sickling due to sickle cell hemoglobin (Hbs) concentration. DRBCs in sickle cell disease patients caused priapism, renal dysfunction, skin ulcer, deletion of α-thalassemia, hyperbilirubinemia, and increased lactate dehydrogenase [38]. There is comorbidity of SCD and malaria among indigenes of Northwestern Nigeria with highest incidence of SS (51.8%), SC (28.4%), AS (16.2%), and SS + F (3.6%), respectively. Hemophilia, epistaxis, and splenomegaly, among others, are associated with SCD. Weight, packed cell volume, hemoglobin, total blood volume, red blood cell volume, and plasma volume are seriously affected in sickle cell patients that are not therapeutically managed causing the need for blood transfusion. Good prognosis is guaranteed by polypharmacy that involves the use of hematonic, anti-sickling, analgesic, antimalarial, and anti-inflammatory drugs. Patients from Northwestern Nigeria can live up to 49 years [24]. *Raphanus sativus*, *Arbutus unedo*, *Luffa acutangula*, *Lycopersicum esculentum*, *Cucumis melo*, *Brassica oleracea* var. capitata, *Allium porrum*, *Petroselinum sativum*, *Phoenix dactylifera*, and *Ficus carica* can be used for management of blood and blood-related diseases including the diseases of erythrocytes [39, 40]. Efforts made toward antimalarial vaccine may be much near to fruition [35].

Autoimmune hemolytic anemia is associated with erythrocytes characterized by hemolysis and autoantibodies of anti-erythrocytes. Neurological sign is common in pernicious anemia. However normal morphology of erythrocytes and leucocytes is necessary for diagnosis of idiopathic thrombocytopenic purpura. But pernicious anemia is characterized by dyserythropoiesis and low vitamin B12 with anti-intrinsic factor and anti-gastric mural cell antibodies being positive. Hence pernicious anemia is treated using vitamin B12 [41]. Complete blood count (CBC) identifies anemia, thrombocytopenia, leukopenia, polycythemia, thrombocytosis, and leukocytosis, but 10–20% of results are abnormal [42].

The life span of erythrocytes in human is 120 days; 20 μl of the erythrocytes are produced daily. But the circulating red blood cells vary among individuals of the same age and gender by over 10%. Mechanisms of anemia in solid tumors are by intrinsic or iatrogenic blood loss; iron or folic acid deficiency; autoimmune, traumatic, or drug-induced hemolysis; bone marrow factor caused by myelofibrosis; marrow necrosis; infection; inflammation; and cancer elsewhere in the body. Erythropoietin is important in the production of erythrocytes. Erythropoietin maybe impaired by tumor inflammatory cytokines [43]. Erythrocytes and hemoglobin promote tumor cell growth by increasing nucleotide-binding oligomerization domain-like receptors' expression and cause induction of IL-1b release, macrophage recruitment, and polarization. Therefore, hemorrhage could be used as a sign of therapeutic failure in cancer patients, because it promotes tumor cell growth and anticancer drug resistance [44]. Facilitation of breast cancer treatment by nano-scaled erythrocytes is via a combination of photodynamic, photothermal, and chemotherapy [45]. Erythrocytes can be lost in the blood lost from cancer surgery and anticancer drugs which affect fast-dividing normal cells and cancerous cells, indicating the drugs cannot differentiate good cells from bad cells [41].

Low calcium concentrations were reported in erythrocytes of patients with depressive disorders [46] indicating that erythrocytes could be used to assess therapeutic success of depressive illness and high calcium level could abate the disease. There was higher concentration of soluble catechol-O-methyltransferase (COMT) in erythrocytes of patients suffering from bulimia nervosa and binge eating disorder than anorexia nervosa [47] indicating that erythrocytes could be used for diagnosis of eating disorders. Favism, neonatal icterus, hereditary non-spherocytic hemolytic anemia, drug-induced hemolytic anemia, and hemolytic anemia due to infection are caused by increased destruction of erythrocytes with enzyme deficiencies. Quinine, chloroquine, sulfadiazine, phenytoin, isoniazid, chloramphenicol, ascorbic acid, and colchicine, among others, could be given in therapeutic doses to G-6-PD-deficient patients without non-spherocytic hemolytic anemia [48]. Hereditary spherocytosis, hereditary elliptocytosis, hereditary pyropoikilocytosis, and hereditary stomatocytosis are hemolytic anemias characterized by heterogeneity and treated by splenectomy which in turn causes complications of cardiovascular diseases, thromboembolic disorders, pulmonary hypertension, and penicillin-resistant pneumococci [49]. Human erythrocytes are subject to degree of genetic diversity. This variability results in anemia, cyanosis, polycythemia, non-hematologic alterations, sickling disorders, unstable hemoglobinopathies, or hemoglobinopathies associated with polycythemia, methemoglobinemia, and α- and β-thalassemias [48]. The cardiovascular effects of SCD and thalassemia are due to iron accumulation and hypoxia, respectively. The risk of thromboembolism should be assessed after splenectomy in the case of congenital chronic hemolytic anemia [50].

Autoimmune hemolytic anemia (AIHA) is potentially severe, characterized by destruction of RBCs and immunoglobulin G (IgG) anti-RBC [51]. Hence, RBC membrane could be used to diagnose autism spectrum disorders using biophotonics [52]. Therefore, relative deformability difference between tumor cells and blood cells as indicated by the length of time [53] may be used to diagnose and determine prognosis of some erythrocyte-related diseases and therapeutic interventions. Small intestinal resection and anastomosis by 70% decreased RBC from 6.23 to 5.1% pre-administration of glutamine. However, RBC decreased from 5.8 to 4.5% on the 12th day of experimentation. Honey, ascorbic acid, and glutamine caused decreased erythrocytes in intestinal resection and anastomosis in dogs [54]. Canine parvoviral enteritis causes anemia with highest incidence in Nigerian local dog occurring in January of every year and prevalence of 5.7% for the past 7 years [55]. Erythrocyte sedimentation is the speed with which erythrocyte levels fall in the blood of normal animals over a period of time. Hence diseased animals have high ESR, whereas healthy animals have low ESR [56] signifying that erythrocyte diseases can be diagnosed using ESR.

4.3 Effects of toxic agents on erythrocytes

Potassium permanganate (16 mg/kg) decreased hematocrit from 41.00 ± 2.08 to $39.29 \pm 2.43\%$ with attendant hypochloremia [16]. Salinity increased hematocrit and decreased hemoglobin of juvenile Nile tilapia (*Oreochromis niloticus*) [57]. Hypertonic saline (20%) could decrease hematocrit, total protein, and albumin [58] invariably decreasing erythrocytes and perhaps increasing hemoglobin. Toxic agents such as plants, drugs, venoms, antivenoms, chemicals, uroliths, and some food additives could damage erythrocytes and consequently cause anemia [59, 61]. Halofantrine, sulfadimidine, chloramphenicol, and other many drugs and chemicals are toxic to erythrocytes [10, 15, 62]. But erythrocytes decreased in Baladi goat during the last 3 weeks of parturition and remained low 2 weeks after parturition [63] perhaps due to significant blood loss.

4.4 Effects of therapeutic agents on erythrocytes

Hexavalent chromium increased erythrocytes from 1.3 ± 0.03 to $1.05 \pm 0.05 \times 10^6\ /\mu l$ after 24 h in *Labeo rohita* (Indian Major Carp), whereas hemoglobin was increased from 8.1 ± 6.7 to 6.80 ± 0.96 g/dl in the same species of animal. Also total protein of gill was decreased from 192.79 ± 4.08 to 171.78 ± 3.64 g/dl [19] suggesting that hexavalent chromium has effect on gill protein. But RBCs of marine teleost carnivorous fish, *Lates calcarifer* ($2.96 \pm 0.25 \times 10^6/\mu l$), are higher than that of omnivorous *Mugil cephalus* ($2.52 \pm 0.21 \times 10^6/\mu l$) and herbivorous *Chanos chanos* ($2.0 \pm 0.51\times 10^6/\mu l$), respectively. But hemoglobin and hematocrit were higher in *L. calcarifer* than in *M. cephalus*, and total protein was also higher in *L. calcarifer* [22]. RBCs of male *Naja naja* ($0.58 \pm 0.04 \times 10^6$/μl) are higher than that of the female *Naja naja* ($0.50 \pm 0.04 \times 10^6$/μl). PCV of the male (30.11 ± 1.93%) is higher than that of the female (23.41 ± 1.67%), whereas hemoglobin (7.6 ± 0.75 g/dl) is significantly higher in male than in the female *Naja naja* (3.25 ± 0.74 g/dl), respectively [64]. The difference in the hematological parameters may be due to their nutrition, age, sex, and environment. Aqueous extract of *Abrus precatorius* seed decreased erythrocytes from 6.33 ± 0.2 to $5.33 \pm 0.24 \times 10^6/\mu l$, packed cell volume from 38.00 ± 1.22 to 32.00 ± 1.41%, and hemoglobin from 12.65 ± 0.9 to 10.68 ± 0.47 g/dl, respectively. Distemper-hepatitis-leptospirosis-parvovirus-parainfluenza (DHLPPi) vaccine decreased in dog, hematological parameters at dose level of >2 mg/kg body weight. The same dose of the extract and DHLPPi caused hypoalbuminemia and hypoglobulinemia and decreased total albumin-globulin ratio. Hence the two could be used in prevention of chronic viral infection in dogs [13], signifying that erythrocytes have relationship with plasma proteins and may be used to determine immune status of animals. Methanol and ethanol seed extract of *Abrus precatorius* decreased erythrocytes from 9.60 ± 1.02 to $7.13 \pm 0.34 \times 10^6/\mu l$ and $6.37 \pm 0.60 \times 10^6/\mu l$, respectively [14], indicating that the plant has anti-erythrocytic principle. Erythrocytes of albino rats increased from 7.2 $\pm 0.14 \times 10^{12}$/L to $9.35 \pm 0.08 \times 10^{12}$/L. Packed cell volume, hemoglobin, and albumin were also increased significantly by aqueous ethanolic extract of *Psidium guajava* [17]. *Escherichia coli* caused hemolysis in *Rattus norvegicus* that was attenuated by aqueous root back extract of *Byrsocarpus coccineus*. *E. coli* was eliminated from the intestine and other organs by the extract [65]. *Chinchilla chinchilla* breed of the rabbit had increased erythrocytes, PCV, and hemoglobin as compared with other breeds [66]. *Vernonia amygdalina* and *Carica papaya* showed significant decrease in *P. berghei* parasites and increased RBCs and hematocrit in mice [67].

But *Ficus thonningii* aqueous extract has ameliorative activity against osmotic fragility induced by acetaminophen [68]. Various extracts of *A. precatorius* showed activity against parasites of erythrocytes such as *Plasmodium*, *Leishmania*, and *Trypanosoma* species with $1C_{50}$ of 12.1 ± 4.59 μg/ml [69]. Ceftriaxone caused increased packed cell volume, hypobilirubinemia, and increased bicarbonate ions in turkeys [15]. However human equivalent dose (HED) formula could be modified for determination of hematological and biochemical parameters [70]. About 8% of body weight correlates very well with plasma cell volume and hematocrit [2]. But many varieties of body surface area formulas could also yield different values of erythrocytes. Wang et al.'s formula may provide moderate doses of anticancer drugs against blood cell cancers [71]. Aqueous leaf extract of *A. precatorius* cleared significant percent of *Plasmodium berghei* in 14 days. However 10^7, *P. berghei* appeared in erythrocytes of mice within 24 hr after intraperitoneal inoculation [62]. Hence the percent of parasitized erythrocytes is calculated as follows:

$$\text{The percentage parasitized} = \frac{\text{Number of infected erythrocytes x 100}}{\text{Number of total erythrocytes}} \tag{3}$$

$$\text{Number of parasites per microliter } (\mu\text{l}) \text{ of blood}$$
$$= \frac{\text{WBC} \times \text{parasites counted against 100 WBC}}{100} \tag{4}$$

Erythrocytes infected with 10^7 *P. berghei* decreased in 7 days by 19%, after inoculation. But aqueous extract of *A. precatorius* leaf and halofantrine caused 9.8 and 12.7% decrease in parasitemia, respectively. However mice-fed grower's marsh had erythrocyte increase of 6.7% in 7 days [62]. The administration of aqueous leaf extract of *A. precatorius* at 10 mg/kg i.p. caused increased hematocrit from 33.0 ± 4.1 to $40.5 \pm 3.1\%$ as compared to 50 mg/kg oral dose that caused $40.3 \pm 3.6\%$, respectively [72]. Gender, age, cholesterol, triglycerides, apoliprotein, and albumin affect hematological parameters [73]. Woman's blood has more fluid with 20% fewer erythrocytes than man's blood. Hence there is less supply of oxygen to body tissues in woman, and therefore she gets tired easily and is more prone to fainting [74]. But hot water increases blood supply to the muscle; hence water is contraindicated in acute bleeding [75].

4.5 Relationship between body weight, body surface area, erythrocytes, and area under curve

Formulas have been derived from the existing formulas that could be used for calculation of body weight, blood volume, erythrocyte volume, and PCV. The derived formulas are:

$$\text{Total blood volume (TBV)} = 0.08\text{BW} \tag{5}$$

$$\text{TBV} = \text{Plasma volume (PV)} \times \frac{100}{100 - \text{Haematocrit}} \tag{6}$$

$$\text{Haemtocrit (RCV)} = \text{TBV} - \text{PV} \tag{7}$$

Equate Eqs. (5) and (6):

$$\text{TBV} = 0.08\text{ BW} = \text{PV} \times \frac{100}{100 - \mathit{Haematocrit}} \tag{8}$$

$$0.08\text{BW} = \text{PV} \times \frac{100}{100 - \text{Haematocrit}} \tag{9}$$

$$\text{BW} = \text{PV} \times \frac{100}{\frac{100 - \text{Haematocrit}}{0.08}} \tag{10}$$

$$\text{BW} = \text{PV} \times \frac{100}{100 - \mathit{Haematocrit}} \times \frac{1}{0.08} \tag{11}$$

But 0.08 = 8% [2].

$$\text{But creatinine clearance } (\mathit{CrCl}) = \frac{\text{K} \times (140 - \text{age}) \times \text{BW}}{\text{D} \times \text{Scr} \times 72} \tag{12}$$

Substitute BW of Eq. (11) in Eq. (12):

$$\text{Hence } \mathit{CrCl} = \frac{K \times (140 - \mathit{age}) \times PV \times \frac{100}{100 - \mathit{Haematocrit}} \times \frac{1}{0.08}}{\text{D x Scr x 72}} \tag{13}$$

$$\text{But serum creatinine (Scr)} = \frac{\mathit{Pcr}}{1440} \times 1000\text{ ml} \tag{14}$$

$$\text{U}_{\text{cr}} = \text{urine creatinine; Pcr} = \text{plasma creatinine}$$

$$\text{D (Depuration)} = \frac{\text{Ucr}}{\text{Pcr}} \tag{15}$$

$$\text{Dose (D)} = \text{AUC} \times [CrCl + 25] \tag{16}$$

where D = dose of either therapeutic agent or toxicant that has an effect on erythrocytes, blood volume, and plasma volume and AUC = area under curve.

However, pharmacokinetic data are more useful in relation to disease of pathological findings instead of focusing on the mean data in relation to risk assessment [76]. Baseline variable is important to consider when using AUC for determination of relevant parameters [77]:

$$\text{Creatinine half} - \text{life}\left(Crt\ \frac{1}{2}\right) = \frac{14616.8}{P_{CL-25}} \tag{17}$$

where P_{CL} = plasma clearance.

$$\text{Metabolism constant (Km)} = \frac{\text{BW}}{\text{BSA}} \tag{18}$$

$$\text{BW} = \text{Km} \times \text{BSA} \tag{19}$$

where BSA = body surface area [78].

However toxic agent could cause lethality by destroying erythrocytes. The amount of a toxicant that causes death in 50% of test animals is called median lethal dose (LD_{50}). The formula is used for determination of both median lethal and median effective dose of snake venom and antivenom, respectively:

$$\therefore \text{LD}_{50} = \frac{\text{ED}_{50}}{3} \times \text{BW} \times 10^{-4} \tag{20}$$

where LD_{50} = median lethal dose of toxic agent that has an effect on erythrocytes of 50% of test animals, ED_{50} = dose that has therapeutic effect on 50% of test animals, and 10^{-4}= safety factor [79].

Substitute BW of Eq. (19) in Eq. (20):

$$\text{Hence LD}_{50} = \frac{\text{ED}_{50}}{3} \times Km \times BSA \times 10^{-4} \tag{21}$$

Equations (18)–(21) are relevant in the study using experimental animals. However, there are various human body surface area formulas that vary from race to race and could be used in calculation of body surface area [80]. But the unique body surface area formula for human and dog may be relevant [81], and it is given below:

$$\text{BSA} = \text{BW}^{0.528} \times \text{H}^{0.528} \times \text{K (where K} = \text{constant} = 0.14) \tag{22}$$

The height of dog must be multiplied by 2, and it is always in meter. More so Treeing Walker Coonhound (65 kg), female Komondor (59 kg), Greater Swiss mountain dog (59 kg), French Mastiff (50 kg), and long-haired St. Bernard (55 kg) have the same body surface area of humans weighing 51.3, 59, 46.7, 44, and 44.8 kg, respectively [81], and the two may have the same erythrocytes and other hematological values. Also, malignant lymphoma (cancer of the white blood cells) and other blood-related cancers can be treated using some other established BSA formulas [80]. But, scorpion sting can cause bleeding, leading to anemia and death. Hence the formula for determination of median lethal dose (LD_{50}) of scorpion venom in experimental animals is given below [82]:

$$\text{LD}_{50} = \text{ED}_{50}^{1/3} \times \text{BW} \times 10^{-4} \tag{23}$$

4.6 Transport of oxygen by erythrocytes

Erythrocytes in contact with alveoli receive oxygen which is combined with hemoglobin (oxyhemoglobin) and transported to various parts of the body. After the delivery of oxygen, the erythrocytes return CO_2 combined with hemoglobin (deoxyhemoglobin) which is bluish in color to the alveoli for expiration. Hence the following reaction occurs in the erythrocytes:

$$H_2O + CO_2 \rightleftharpoons H_2CO_3 \rightleftharpoons H^+ + HCO_3^- \rightleftharpoons H_2O + CO_2 \quad (24)$$

The presence of COOH and C=O in piroxicam and other chemically related compounds [83] may interfere with chemistry of erythrocytes causing hemolysis and anemia. Also degradation products of some polymers, poly(lactic-co-glycolic acid), polyethylene glycol, polycaprolactone, and poly(propylene glycol) are converted to lactic acid and glycolic acid which are in turn converted to carbon dioxide and water [84] indicating that some polymers could also affect erythrocytes. Polycythemia could be confirmed by hyperpnea. Meat from an animal poisoned with potassium permanganate could react with 0.2% ethanolic benzidine changing the color of meat to dark green in 1–2 s [85], and potassium permanganate causes hyperpnea. Lowest oxygen saturation could be improved by zolpidem [86]. Erythrocytes of cow, dog, goat, horse, pig, rabbit, rat, and sheep composed greatly of cholesterol and cholesteryl esters, triglycerides, and free fatty acids are present in trace quantity. They may not be true constituents of erythrocytes, but rather contaminants from plasma lipoproteins or leucocytes. Cholesterol is 30% of cell lipid and has molar ratio with phospholipid [87] and may affect oxygen capacity of erythrocytes. Hence cow, sheep, horse, rabbit, and chicken erythrocytes are susceptible to *Vibrio vulnificus* hemolysin with varying degrees of susceptibility [88] and may cause anemia and less oxygen transport. Human coagulation factor 1X (F-1X) activated by human RBCs causes coagulation activated by enzyme in the RBC membrane. However, in dog, cattle, rabbit, and sheep, coagulation did not occur except in pig when procoagulant was used. Hence coagulation activation of enzyme may be present in these species of animals [89].

Lysis of erythrocytes by toxins of cobra could cause anemia and splitting of phospholipids in equal capacity in rabbit, dog, human, and guinea pig, but not in camel and sheep erythrocytes. Phosphatide acylhydrolase is responsible for splitting of the erythrocytes. The action is via lytic factor which is hemolytic. The phospholipase readily hydrolyzes phospholipids of erythrocytes. *Vipera palestinae* could not lyse erythrocytes and hydrolyze phospholipids [90]. Plasma viscosity depends on plasma protein concentration [91], with cattle having 1.72 mpa s and rabbit (1.3 mpa s) with horse, dog, cat, mouse, rat, pig, and sheep having 1.3–1.7 mpa s. Man has a value lower than this range [92]. Deformability of RBCs is dependent on size and shape [93] with pig, hamster, rat, mouse, and rabbit having more deformable RBCs than sheep, horse, elephant, and dog. The deformity is characterized by RBC elongation and aggregation [94]. All these could affect oxygen transport. Non-irreversible sickle cells adhere more at normal oxygen tension, and more than 1% of the cells remained adhered to the monolayer at forces higher than physiologic shear stresses [95].

4.7 Morphologic differences in erythrocytes of animals

Llama, dromedary, and camel have low hematocrit value and low RBC aggregation [96]. Such RBCs may be small and elliptical in shape [97]. Nonmammalian RBCs have nucleus and microtubular bundle connected to a marginal band [98].

The erythrocytes are elliptical, larger, and not bending, with decreased blood cell count. But nonnucleated erythrocytes exhibit nonalignment. Hence erythrocytes of bird are flattened, lenticular, spherical, and folded when deformed [99]. Hemoglobin concentration of nonmammalian erythrocytes is 15–20% higher than that of mammalian species, with increased RBC density, and the nucleus contains 20% of cytoplasmic volume [100, 101] with RBC rigidity [102]. However, RBCs of reptiles are least decreased than that of mammal, the membrane having shear elastic modulus [103]. But fish might have the largest RBC volumes. The cells are elliptical and bulge in the region of their nucleus. Fish hematocrit drops with water temperature and can change due to the environmental temperature [104]. Aggregation capacity of equine erythrocyte is higher than that of dog and sheep, but could not be measured. There is species variation in erythrocyte elongation not linked with the aggregation property. Also deformability of erythrocytes is species-specific [105]. Tannic acid increases or decreases agglutinability of erythrocytes in the presence of immune serum [106]. Attachment of endotoxins, e.g., lipopolysaccharide antigen, to erythrocytes was strongly prevented by mammalian and avian sera followed by that of reptilian (moderate) and amphibian (minimal) [107]. But temperature has no effect on flexibility of horse, cattle, sheep, goat, and some human erythrocytes indicating that blood viscosity varies with temperature [108]. Diameter, circumference, and surface area are higher in erythrocytes of dog followed by horse, cattle, sheep, and goat in that order [109].

4.8 Metabolic pathway of erythrocytes

Ion transport pathways of the erythrocytes are $Na^+ - K^+ - Cl^-$, $Na^+ - Cl^-$, and $Na^+ - K^+$ through AQPI water and SKI− Gardos channels using ATPase [110]. Major metabolic pathway in erythrocytes is as follows: glucose is converted to glucose-6-phosphate to fructose-6-phosphate to pyruvate to lactate [111]. Reduced or defective erythrocytes result in nonregenerative anemia, and increased cell loss results in regenerative anemia, respectively [112]. Cellular shape and flexibility of erythrocytes are dependent on metabolic process which is via enzymes that are associated with erythrocyte defects [113]. Spherocytes have less diameter and thickness greater than normal resulting from hereditary spherocytosis seen in the peripheral blood smear of neonates with ABO incompatibility [114], releasing lipids, causing adenosine triphosphate depletion, and exposing the cells to shear stress [115]. Methods used for measurements of erythrocytes deformability are filtration microfluidic filtration and laser diffractometry. Deformation of RBCs has to do with the geometry, hemoglobin concentration, rheological properties, osmotic concentration, calcium, nitric oxide, temperature, membrane protein and lipid alteration, erythrocyte ATP, and erythrocyte aging. But measurements of individual cells are by micropipette aspiration, atomic force microscopy, optical tweezers, and quantitative phase imaging. Also, there is correlation between erythrocyte deformability and diabetic microangiopathy [116]. Eosin-5-maleimide (EMA) binding test and osmotic fragility test differentiate hereditary spherocytosis from hereditary stomatocytosis [117]. Morphological changes in the sickle cell hemoglobin caused by deoxygenation of RBCs could lead to high metabolic activity and shortened life span of erythrocytes in sickle cell disease patients [118] invariably leading to anemia. The mechanism extent, levels, and complement involvement differ considerably in autoimmune hemolytic anemia [119]. Erythrocyte membrane disorders including hereditary spherocytosis and elliptocytosis could be diagnosed by red blood cell cytology, ektacytometry, flow cytometry, electrophoresis, and mutational analysis of cell membrane proteins [120].

4.9 Anemia as a major sign of erythrocyte deformation

Causes of anemia in cats are acute blood loss, chronic inflammatory disease, renal disease, feline leukemia, immune-mediated hemolytic anemia, pure red cell aplasia, myeloproliferative syndrome, mycoplasma infection, cytauxzoonosis, iron deficiency, and nutritional deficiency. The prognosis of feline nonregenerative anemia is variable, reversible, chronic, or fatal [121]. The spleen contributes to anemia by removing the damaged erythrocytes. Hereditary spherocytosis is spectrin-deficient and ankyrin-deficient erythrocytes dependent and could cause hemolysis [122]. Glycogen storage disease could affect erythrocytes. The disease is classified as follows: Type 1 (von Gierke's disease) is caused by deficiency of glucose-6-phosphate, whereas type 2 (Pompe's disease) is generalized glycogenosis. But type 3 (limit dextrinosis) is characterized by deficiency of the amylo-1, 6-glucosidase or debrancher enzyme, and type 4 is characterized by hepatic cirrhosis, abnormal glycogen resembling amylopectin, and deficiency of amylo-1, 4-1, 6-transglucosidase. Type 5 is characterized by weakness of muscle and phosphorylase deficiency in adults, and type 6 is clinically similar to type 1, characterized by higher phosphorylase. But type 3 has the highest concentration of glycogen, in the erythrocytes, but the concentration of glycogen is normal in type 1 and 2 [123].

Plasmodium species, *Babesia* species, and Bartonella species can target erythrocytes directly, whereas immunogens, microbial toxins, crypt antigens, and suppression of erythropoiesis can target erythrocytes indirectly. Duffy blood group antigens, ABO blood group antigens, Knops blood group antigen, Gerbich blood group antigen, babesiosis, bartonellosis, and toxoplasmosis target RBCs primarily. Erythrocytes are targeted for immunogenic clearance of *Mycoplasma pneumoniae*, *Haemophilus influenzae* type B, *Salmonella* species, polyagglutination T activation, *Clostridium perfringens*, parvovirus B19, Epstein-Barr virus, and acquired B antigen [124]. Disorders of erythrocytes hydration are overhydration, hereditary hydrocytosis, cryohydrocytosis, dehydration, and hereditary xerocytosis which are genetic [125]. Chronic liver disease could cause anemia but requires a complex diagnostic approach [126]. Hereditary erythrocyte volume homeostasis is heterogeneous with phenotypes ranging from overhydrated to dehydrated erythrocytes usually characterized by laboratory, physiological, clinical, and genetic findings [127].

Examination of urine sediment could serve as a guide for diagnosis and management of kidney disease [128] in relation to erythrocyte disorders. Erythrocytes have linked type 2 diabetes and Alzheimer disease in human. Superimposed alterations have been observed in Alzheimer disease patients caused by oxidative stress of erythrocytes [129], suggesting that therapeutic target on RBCs could alleviate Alzheimer disease. Hence erythrocytes' mechanical properties toward microfluidics could provide a clinical correlate in diseases of erythrocytes [130]. End-stage renal disease causes alteration of erythrocytes. Therefore, erythrocytes from peritoneal dialysis patients are more prone to aggregation that may be caused by uremia, hypoproteinemia, and high oxidative stress on erythrocytes, impairing blood flow dynamics and causing inadequate microcirculatory perfusion [131]. Erythrocyte complement receptor type 1 (E-CR 1) level of expression could be used as a diagnostic marker for systemic lupus erythematosus (SLE) [132]. The level of concentration of methotrexate polyglutamate in erythrocytes is associated with alleviation of rheumatoid arthritis [133].

Blood transfusion and febrile condition could also affect morphology of erythrocytes and erythrocyte count [134]. However, 15% of cancer patients with anemia are given blood transfusion and with hemoglobin level of <9 g/dl used as index of anemia. After transfusion hemoglobin rises by 1 g/dl, and the transfused erythrocytes last for 100–110 days with complications including but not limited to iron overload, viral and bacterial infections, immune injury, non-Hodgkin lymphoma, and chronic lymphocytic leukemia which are some worst outcome in selected cancers [135]. Trypanosomosis, pediculosis, helminthosis, lousiness, colibacillosis, babesiosis, coccidiosis, and amoebiasis characterized by anemia in advanced condition could be treated using various species of medicinal plants. The therapeutic principles are alkaloids, tannins, saponins, glycosides, flavonoids, phenols, minerals, and vitamins [136]. Health education could lead to disappearing of blood-related diseases such as malaria [137]. Ebola affects the blood leading to hemorrhage, septic shock, and multiple organ failure [138]. This point to the need for transfusion which could not be instituted until blood and erythrocytes are assessed. Because less than 1% dense hematocrit could cause aneurysm in aged dogs, canine hematocrit is an accurate model for human hematocrit [139].

5. Conclusion

Erythrocytes are red blood cells that transport oxygen from the alveoli to other parts of the body. Hence they are very vital connective tissues that play a metabolic role on the functional organ system. Its pathological features could be used for diagnosis of a myriad of metabolic, non-metabolic, infectious, noninfectious, hereditary, and non-hereditary diseases. Erythrocyte shape, size, area, and volume could be used to determine a prognosis of a disease. Erythrocytes also store some drugs invariably prolonging their half-life. Hemolysis can lead to anemia that is treated using hematonics. But severe blood loss is corrected by blood transfusion.

Author details

Saganuwan Alhaji Saganuwan
Federal University of Agriculture Makurdi, Nigeria

*Address all correspondence to: pharn_saga2006@yahoo.com

References

[1] Shier D, Butler J, Lewis R. Hole's Essential of Human Anatomy and Physiology. New York: McGraw-Hill; 2006. p. 590

[2] Saganuwan SA, Onyeyili PA. Haematonic and plasma expander effects of aqueous leaf extract of *Abrus precatorius* in *Mus musculus*. Comparative Clinical Pathology. 2012; **21**(6):1249-1255

[3] Seeley RR, Stephens TD, Tate P. Anatomy and Physiology. 6th ed. New York: McGraw-Hill; 2003. p. 1105

[4] Ganong FW. Review of Medical Physiology. 21st ed. New York: McGraw-Hill; 2003. p. 912

[5] Brown BA. Haematology Principles and Procedures. 2nd ed. Philadelphia: Lea and Febiger; 1976. pp. 56-81

[6] Crowley LV. Anaemia. In: Crowley LV, editor. An Introduction to Human Disease, Pathology and Pathophysiology Correlations. 5th ed. Sudbury: Jones & Bartlett; 2001. p. 790

[7] Porth CM. Pathophysiology, Concepts of Altered Health States. 3rd ed. Vol. 1158. Philadelphia: JB Lippincott; 1992

[8] Lawlor GJ, Fisher TJ. Manual of Allergy and Immunology: Diagnosis and Therapy. 2nd ed. Boston: Little Brown and Company; 1989. p. 511

[9] Kahn CM. The Merck Veterinary Manual. 9th ed. Whitehouse Station: Merck & Co, Inc; 2005. p. 2712

[10] Tripath KD. Essentials of Medical Pharmacology. 5th ed. New Delhi: Jaypee Brothers Medical Publishers; 2004. p. 875

[11] Brooks GA, Fahey TD, White TP, Baldwin KM. Exercise Physiology: Human Biogenetics and Its Applications. 3rd ed. New-York: McGraw-Hill; 2008. p. 851

[12] Seeley RR, Stephens TD, Tate P. Anatomy and Physiology. 2nd ed. St. Louis: Mosby; 1992. p. 98

[13] Tion MT, Fotina HA, Saganuwan A. Comparative haematological and biochemical effects of cocktail vaccine (DHLLP;) and *Abrus precatorius* seed aqueous extract on canine parvoviral vaccinated and unvaccinated Nigerian local dogs. Scientific Messenger LNUVMB. 2018;**20**(92):1-6

[14] Tion MT, Fotina H, Saganuwan SA. Phytochemical screening, proximate analysis, median lethal dose (LDSO), haematological and biochemical effects of various extracts of *Abrus precatorius* seeds in *Mus musculus*. JAVAR. 2018; **5**(3):354-360

[15] Saganuwan SA. Effects of ceftriaxone on haematological and biochemical parameters of Turkey. ARI. 2006;**3**(3):562-565

[16] Saganuwan SA, Ahur VM, Yohanna CA. Acute toxicity studies of potassium permanganate in Swiss albino mice. Nigerian Journal of Physiological Sciences. 2008;**23**(1–2):31-35

[17] Adamu AS. Effects of aqueous-ethanolic extract of guava (*Psidium guajava* linn) leaves on reproductive functions of albino rats [MSc thesis]. Nigeria: Federal University of Agriculture Makurdi; 2017

[18] Daramola JO, Adetoye AA, Fatoba TA, Soladoye AO. Haematological and biochemical parameters of West African dwarf goats. Livestock Research for Rural Development. 2005;**17**(8):1-9

[19] Vutukuru SS. Acute effects of hexavalent chromium on survival,

oxygen consumption, haematolgoical parameters and some biochemical profiles of the Indian Major Carp, Labeo rohita. International Journal of Environmental Research and Public Health. 2005;**2**(3):456-462

[20] Durgun Z, Keskin E, Atalay B. Selected haematological and biochemical values in ostrich chicks and growers. Archive Geflugelkd. 2005; **59**(2):62-66

[21] Azeez OI, Oyagbemi AA, Olawuwo OS, Oyewale JO. Changes in haematology, plasma biochemistry and erythrocyte osmotic fragility of the Nigerian laughing dove (*Streptopelia senegalensis*) in captivity. Nigerian Journal of Physiological Sciences. 2013; **28**:63-68

[22] Satheeshkumar P, Ananthan G, Kumar DS, Jagadeesan L. Haematology and biochemical parameters of different feeding behaviour of teleost fishes from Vellar estuary, India. Comparative Clinical Pathology. 2010;**21**(6):1-5. DOI: 10.1007 500580-011-1259-7

[23] Coroian CO, Miresan V, Coroian A, Raducu C, Andronie L, Marchis Z, et al. Biochemical and haematological blood parameters at different stages of lactations in cows. Bulletin of University of Agricultural Sciences and Veterinary Medicine. Animal Science and Biotechnologies. 2017;**74**(1):31-36

[24] Saganuwan SA. The pattern of sickle cell disease in sickle cell patients from Northwestern Nigeria. Clinical Medicine Insights: Therapeutics. 2016;**8**:53-57

[25] Kumar V, Cotran RS, Robbins SL. Robbins Basic Pathology. 7th ed. Canada: Saunders, An Imprint of Elsevier; 2003. p. 873

[26] Arikan H, Cicek K. Haematology of amphibians and reptiles: A review. North-Western Journal of Zoology. 2014;**10**(1):190-209

[27] Jenkins-Perez J. Hematologic Evaluation of Reptiles: A Diagnostic Mainstay. Veterinary Technician; 2012: E1-E8

[28] Dal' Bo GA, Sampaio FG, Losekann ME, de Queiroz JF, Luiz AJB, Wolf VHG, et al. Hematological and morphometric blood value of our cultured species of economically important tropical food fish. Neotropical Ichthyology. 2015;**13**(2): 439-446

[29] Njidda AA, Hassan IT, Olatunji EA. Haematological and biochemical parameters of goats of semi-Arid environment fed on natural grazing rangeland of Northern Nigeria. IOSR Journal of Agriculture and Veterinary Science. 2013;**3**(2):01-08

[30] Radkowska I, Herbut E. Haematological and biochemical blood parameters in dairy cows depending on the management system. Animal Science Papers and Reports. 2014;**32**(4): 317-325

[31] Fazio F, Marafioti S, Arfuso F, Ficcione G, Faggio C. Comparative study of the biochemical and haematological parameters of wild Tyrrhenian fish species. Veterinary Medicine. 2013;**11**:576-581

[32] Njidda AA, Shuaibu AA, Isidahomen CE. Haematological and serum biochemical indices of sheep in semi-arid environment of northern Nigeria. Global Journal of Science Frontier Research. 2014;**14**(2):1-9

[33] Etim NAN, Williams NE, Akpabio U, Offiong EFA. Haematological parameters and factors affecting their values. Agricultural Sciences. 2014;**2**(1): 37-47

[34] Mauricio CRM, Schneider FK, Takahira RK, Santos LC, Gamba HR. Image-based red blood cell counter for multiple species of wild and domestic

animals. Arquivo Brasileiro de Medicina Veterinária e Zootecnia (ABMVZ). 2017;**69**(1):75-84

[35] Saganuwan SA, Onyeyti PA. Malaria and its therapeutic implications: The way forward. International Journal of Tropical Disease & Health. 2014;**4**(7): 802-840

[36] Saganuwan SA, Yatswako S. Malaria parasites of clinical and laboratory importance—An update. Journal of Medical and Pharmaceutical Sciences. 2006;**2**(3):36-40

[37] Kimura M, Teramoto I, Chan CW, Idris ZM, Kongere J, Kagaya W, et al. Improvement of malaria diagnostic system based on acridine orange staining. Malaria Journal. 2018; **17**(72):1-6

[38] Bartolucci P, Brugnara C, Teixeira-Pinto A, Pissard S, Moradkham K, Jovult H, et al. Erythrocyte density in sickle cell syndromes is associated with specific clinical manifestations and hemolysis. Blood. 2012;**120**(15): 3136-3141. DOI: 10.1182/blood-2012-04-424184

[39] Saganuwan SA. Some medicinal plants of Arabian Peninsula. Journal of Medicinal Plant Research: Planta Medica. 2010;**4**(9):766-788

[40] Saganuwan SA. A photo album of some medicinal plants of the Nigerian middle belt. Journal of Herbs, Spices & Medicinal Plants. 2010;**16**(3):219-292

[41] Yokoyama K, Ikeda Y. Autoimmune hematological diseases. JMAJ. 2004; **47**(9):412-418

[42] Teferi A, Hanson CA, Inwards DJ. How to interpret and pursue an abnormal complete blood cell count in adults. Mayo Clinic Proceedings. 2005; **80**(7):923-936

[43] Spivak JL. Cancer-related anaemia: Its causes and characteristics. Seminars in Oncology. 1994;**21**(3):3-8

[44] Tin T, He S, Liu X, Jiang W, Ye Y, Lin Z, et al. Extracellular red blood cells and hemoglobin promote tumor growth and therapeutic resistance as endogenous danger signals. Journal of Immunology. 2015;**194**:429-437

[45] Wan G, Chen B, Li L, Wang D, Shi S, Zhang D, et al. Nanoscaled red blood cells facilitate breast cancer treatment by combining photothermal/photodynamic therapy and chemotherapy. Biomalerial. 2018;**155**:25-40

[46] Kamei K, Tabata O, Muneoka K, Muraoka SI, Tomiyoshi R, Takigawa M. Electrolytes in erythrocytes of patients with depressive disorders. Psychiatry and Clinical Neurosciences. 1998;**52**: 529-533

[47] Amorim-Barbosa T, Serrao MP, Brando I, Vieira-Coelho MA. Catechol-O-methyl transferase activity in erythrocytes from patients with eating disorders. Eating and Weight Disorders Studies on Anorexia, Bulimia and Obesity. 2016;**21**(2):221-227

[48] Van Solinge WW, Van Wijk R. Erythrocyte enzyme disorders. In: Kaushansky K, Lichtman MA, Prichal JT, Levi MM, Press OW, Burns LJ, Caligiuri M (eds) William's Hematology, 9th ed., Mc Graw-Hill Education, Minion Pro, 2015:3-2393

[49] Gallagher PG, Jarolim P. Red cell membrane disorders. In: Hoffman R, Furie B, Benz EJ, McGlave P, Silberstein LE, Shattil SJ (eds). Basic Principles and Practice. Philadelphia: Churchill Livingstone; 2009:623-643

[50] Mozos I. Mechanisms linking red blood cell disorders and cardiovascular diseases. BioMed Research International. 2015:1-12

[51] Sonneveld ME, de Haas M, Koeleman C, de Haan N, Zeerleder SS, Ligthart PC, Wuhrer M, van der Schoot CE, Vidarsson G. Patients with IgG 1-anti-red blood cell antibodies show aberrant Fc-glycosylation. Scientific Reports. 2017;7:1-9

[52] Giacometti G, Ferreri C, Sansone A, Chatgilialoglu C, Mazetti C, Spyratou E, et al. High predictive values of RBC membrane-based diagnostics by biophotonics in an integrated approach for autism spectrum disorders. Scientific Reports. 2017;7(1):1-9

[53] Bagnall JS. Deformability of tumor cells versus blood cells. Nature. 2017;**5**: 1-12

[54] Kisani AI, Adeyanju JB, Sonfada ML. Haematological and biochemical changes in Nigerian dogs with short bowel syndrome. World's Veterinary Journal. 2017;7(3):89-100

[55] Tion MT, Apaa TT, Saganuwan SA, Nwanko HC, Tughgba T, Anumtyo TM, et al. The epidemiology of canine parvoviral enteritis in dogs of Makurdi, Benue State, Nigeria. World's Veterinary Journal. 2018;**8**(3):48-54

[56] Coles EH. Veterinary Clinical Pathology. 2nd ed. Philadelphia: WB Saunders Company; 1974. p. 615

[57] Bosisio F, Fernandes K, Rezende FO, Barbieri E. Alterations in the haemotological parameters of juvenile Nile tilapia (*Oreochromis niloticus*) submitted to different salinities. Pan-American Journal of Aquatic Sciences. 2017;**12**(2):146-154

[58] Saganuwan SA, Ahur VM, Mhonga LI. Sodium chloride decrease body weight of non-water deprived *Rattus norvegicus*. Australian Journal of Basic and Applied Sciences. 2010;**4**(8): 322-329

[59] Tion MT, Dvorska J, Saganuwan SA. A review on urolithiasis in dogs and cats. Bulgarian Journal of Veterinary Medicine. 2015;**18**(1):1-18

[60] Saganuwan SA. Toxicity studies of drugs and chemicals in animals: An overview. Bulgarian Journal of Veterinary Medicine. 2017;**20**(4): 291-318

[61] Andrews GS, Simon UT, John AU, Godwin OO, Alexander NI, Ikagu YM. Studies on changes in some haematological and plasma biochemical parameters in Wister rats fed on diets containing calcium carbide ripened mango fruits. International Journal of Food Science and Nutrition Engineering. 2018;**8**(2):27-36

[62] Saganuwan SA, Onyeyili PA, Ameh EG, Etuk EU. In vivo antiplasmodial activity by aqueous extract of Abrus precatorius in mice. Revista Latinoamericana de Química. 2011;**39** (1–2):32-44

[63] Azab ME, Abdel-Maksoud HA. Changes in some haematological and biochemical parameters during prepartum and postpartum period in female Baladi goats. Small Ruminant Research. 1999;**34**(1):77-85

[64] Dissanzayake DSB, Thewarage LD, Rathnayake RMPM, Kularatne AMK, Ranasinghe JGS, Rajapakse PVJ. Hematological and plasma biochemical parameters in a wild population of *Naja naja* (Linnaeus, 1785) in Sri Lanka. Journal of Venomous Animals and Toxins including Tropical Diseases. 2017;**23**(8):1-9

[65] Ejeh AS. Effects of aqueous root bark extract of Byrsocarpus coccineus on castor oil and bacterial induced diarrhea in albino rats (*Rattus norvegicus*) [MSc thesis]. Nigeria: Federal University of Agriculture Makurdi; 2018

[66] Chineke CA, Ologun AG, Ikeobi CON. Haematological parameters in rabbit breeds and crosses in humid tropics. Pakistan Journal of Biological Sciences. 2006;**9**(11):2102-2106

[67] Okpe O, Habila N, Ikwebe J, Upev VA, Okoduwa SIR, Isaac OT. Antimalaria potential of carica papaya and Vernonia amygdalina in mice infected with *Plasmodium berghei*. Journal of Tropical Medicine. 2016:1-6

[68] Ahur VM, Adenkola YA, Saganuwan SA, Ikye-Tor T. Ameliorative properties of aqueous extract of ficus thonningii on erythrocyte osmotic fragility induced by acetaminophen in Rattus norvegicus. Veterinary Research Forum. 2013;**4**(4): 207-212

[69] Saganuwan SA, Onyeyili PA, Ameh IG, Nwodo NJ, Brun R. In vitro antiplasmodial, antitrypanosomal, antileishmanial and cytotoxic activities of various fractions of *Abrus precatorius* leaf. International Journal of Tropical Disease & Health. 2015;**5**(3):221-229

[70] Saganuwan SA. The paradox of human equivalent dose formula: A canonical case study of Abrus precatorius aqueous leaf extract in monogastric animals. Macedonian Veterinary Review. 2016;**39**(1):23-32

[71] Saganuwan SA, Ndakotsu AM. Standardization and scoring of the body surface area (bsa) formula for calculation of the doses of anticancer agents for cancer patients from the North Western Nigeria. Journal of Cancer Science and Therapy. 2015;**7**(1): 012-018

[72] Saganuwan SA, Onyeyili PA, Suleiman AO. Comparative toxicological effects of orally and intraperitoneally administered aqueous extracts of *Abrus precatorius* leaf in *Mus musculus*. Herba Polonica. 2013;**56**(3): 32-44

[73] Wang MC, Huang CE, Lin MH, Yang YHCH, Chen PT, Nu YY, et al. Impacts of demographic and laboratory parameters on key hematological indices in an adult population of Southern-Taiwan; a cohort study. PLoS One. 2018; **13**(8):1-14

[74] Horay P, Harp D. Hot water therapy: How to Save Your Back, Neck and Shoulders in 10 Minutes A Day of Exercise in Your Shower, Bath or Hot Tub. 10th ed. New Delhi: Orient Paperbacks; 2010. p. 150

[75] Smalley G. The Joy of Committed Love: A Handbook for Husband. Vol. 168. India: Better Yourself Books; 2016

[76] Ploemen JPHTM, Kramer H, Krajnc EI, Martin I. The use of toxicokinetic data in periodical safety assessment: A toxicologic pathologist perspective. Toxicologic Pathology. 2007;**35**:834-837

[77] Scheff JD, Almon RR, DuBis DC, Jusko WJ, Androulakis IP. Assessment of pharmacologic area under the curve when baselines are variable. Pharmaceutical Research. 2011;**28**(5): 1081-1089

[78] Saganuwan SA. The use of body surface area for determination of age, body weight, urine creatinine, plasma creatinine, serum creatinine, urine volume, and creatinine clearance; the reliable canonical method of assessing renotoxicity in animals. Comparative Clinical Pathology. 2018;**27**:1531-1536

[79] Saganuwan SA. Calculation of effective dose fifty (ED_{50}) of antivenin for American pit viper venom. Comparative Clinical Pathology. 2018; **27**:1321-1325

[80] Saganuwan SA, Ndakotsu AM. Standardization and scoring of the body surface area (bsa) formulas for calculation of the doses of anticancer agents for cancer patients from the

North-Western Nigeria. Journal of Cancer Science and Therapy. 2015;**7**(1):012-018

[81] Saganuwan SA. Derivation of a unique body surface area (bsa) formula for calculation of relatively safe doses of dog and human anticancer drugs. Journal of Cancer Science and Therapy. 2017;**9**(10):690-704

[82] Saganuwan SA. Determination of median effect dose (ED_{50}) of scorpion antivenom against scorpion envenomation using a newly developed formula. Animal Models and Experimental Medicine. 2008;**1**:228-234

[83] Saganuwan SA. Piroxicam: Source for synthesis of central nervous system (cns) acting drugs. CNSAMC. 2017;**17**(2):1-5

[84] Saganuwan SA. Biomedical application of polymers: A case of non-CNS drugs becoming CNS acting drugs. Central Nervous System Agents in Medicinal Chemistry. 2017;**17**(3):1-7

[85] Balji Y, Adilbekov Z, Scheiko Y, Seidenova S, Ismagulova G, Zamaratskaia G. A rapid and sensitive method to determine potassium permanganate in meat. Journal of Consumer Protection and Food Safety. 2018:1-6

[86] Mickelson SA. Perioperative monitoring in obstructive sleep apnea hypopnea syndrome. In: Sleep Apnea and Snoring. 2009

[87] Nelson GJ. Composition of neural lipids from erythrocytes of common mammals. Journal of Lipid Research. 1967;**8**:374-379

[88] Tamanaka H, Shimatani S, Tanaka M, Katsu T, Ono B, Shinoda S. Susceptibility of erythrocytes from several animal species to Vibrio vulnificus hemolysin. FEMS Microbiology Letters. 1989;**61**:251-256

[89] Kaibara M, Shinozaki T, Kita R, Iwata H, Ujiie H, Sasaki K, et al. Analysis of coagulation of blood in different animal species with special reference to procoagulant species with special reference to procoagulant activity of red blood cells. Journal of Japanese Society of Biorheology. 2006;**20**(1):35-43

[90] Condrea E, Mammon Z, Aloof S, de Vries A. Susceptibility of erythrocytes of various animal species to the hemolytic and phospholipid splitting action of snake venom. Biochimica et Biophysica Acta. 1964;**84**(4):365-375

[91] Kaymaz AA, Tamer S, Albeniz I, Cefle K, Palanduz S, Ozturk S, et al. Alterations in rheological properties and erythrocytes membrane proteins in cats with diabetes mellitus. Clinical Hemorheology and Microcirculation. 2005;**33**:81-88

[92] Windberger U, Bertholovitsch A, Plasenzotti R, Korak KJ, Heinke G. Whole blood viscosity, plasma viscosity and erythrocyte aggregation in nine mammalian species: Reference values and comparison of data. Experimental Physiology. 2003;**88**:431-440

[93] Windberger U, Plasenzotti R, Voracek T. The fluidity of blood in African elephants (*Loxodonta africana*). Clinical Hemorheology and Microcirculation. 2005;**33**:321-326

[94] Windberger U, Ribitsch V, Resch KL, Losert U. The viscoelasticity of blood and plasma in pig, horse, dog and sheep. Journal of Experimental Animal Science. 1993/1994;**36**:89-95

[95] Smith BD, La Celle PL. Erythrocyte-endothelial cell adherence in sickle cell disorders. Blood. 1986;**68**(5):1050-1054

[96] Johnn H, Phipps C, Gascoyne SC, Hawkey C, Rampling MW. A comparison of the viscometric properties of the blood from a wide

range of mammals. Clinical Hemorheology and Microcirculation. 1992;**12**:639-647

[97] Van Houten D, Weiser MG, Johnson L, Garry F. Reference hematologic values and morphologic features of blood cells in healthy adult Llamas. American Journal of Veterinary Research. 1992;**53**:1773-1775

[98] Nikinmaa M. Vertebrate Red Blood Cells. Berlin: Siringer; 1990

[99] Gaehtgens P, Schmidt F, Will G. Comparative rheology of nucleated and non-nucleated red blood cells I. Microrheology of avian erythrocytes during capillary flow. Pflügers Archiv. 1981;**390**:278-282

[100] Hawkey CM, Bennett PM, Gascoyne SC, Hart MG, Kirkwood JK. Erythrocyte size, number and haemoglobin content in vertebrates. British Journal of Haematology. 1991;**77**: 392-397

[101] Nguyen DP, Tamuguchi K, Scheid P, Piiper J. Kinetics of oxygen uptake and release by red blood cells of chicken and duck. The Journal of Experimental Biology. 1986;**125**:15-27

[102] Mirsalimi SM, Julian RJ. Reduced erythrocyte deformability as a possible contributing factor to pulmonary hypertension and ascites in broiler chickens. Avian Diseases. 1992;**33**: 871-877

[103] Waugh RE. Red cell deformability in different vertebrate animals. Clinical Hemorheology and Microcirculation. 1992;**12**:649-656

[104] Nash GB, Egginton S. Comparative theology of human and trout red blood cells. The Journal of Experimental Biology. 1993;**174**:109-122

[105] Plasenzotti R, Stoiber B, Posch M, Windberger U. Red blood cell deformability and aggregation behaviour in different animal species. Clinical Hemorheology and Microcirculation. 2004;**31**:105-111

[106] Garabedian GA. The behaviour of tanned erythrocytes in various haemagglutination systems. Journal of General Microbiology. 1965;**38**: 181-187

[107] Praino M, Neter E. Effect of scrum from various animals species on erythrocytes attachment of endotoxins and other bacterial antigens. Infection and Immunity. 1972;**18**(3):612-616

[108] Amin TM, Sirs JA. The blood rheology of man and various animal species. Quarterly Journal of Experimental Physiology. 1985;**70**:37-49

[109] Adili N, Melizi M, Belabbas H. Species determination using the red blood cells morphometry in domestic animals. Veterinary World. 2016;**9**(9): 960-963

[110] An X, Mohandas N. Disorders of red cell membrane. British Journal of Haematology. 2008;**141**:367-375

[111] Prankerd TAJ. Enzyme assays in diseases of erythrocytes. Journal of Clinical Pathology. 1970;**24**(4):71-74

[112] Villiers E. Disorders of erythrocytes. In: BSAVA Manual of Canine and Feline Clinical Pathol. 3rd ed., 2016:1-624

[113] Tavazzi D, Taher A, Cppellini MD. Red blood cell enzyme disorders: an overview. Pediatric Annals. 2008;**37**(5): 303-310

[114] Bain BJ, Batse I, Caffan MA. Blood cell morphology in health and disease. British Journal of Haematology 2017; **178**(4):652

[115] Gallagher PG. Disorders of erythrocyte hydration. Blood. 2017;**130** (25):2699-2708

[116] Kim J, Lee HY, Shin S. Advances in the measurement of red blood cell deformability. A brief review. Journal of Cellular Biotechnology. 2015;**1**:63-79

[117] King MJ, Zanella A. Hereditary red cell membrane disorders and laboratory diagnostic testing. International Journal of Laboratory Hematology. 2013;**35**(3):237-243

[118] Boyo AE, Ikomi-Kumm JA. Increased metabolic heat production of erythrocytes in sickle-cell disease. Lauret. 1972;**299**(7762):1215-1216

[119] Berentsen S, Sundic T. Red blood cell destruction in autoimmune hemolytic anemia: Role of complement and potential new targets for therapy. BioMed Research International. 2015:1-11

[120] Da Costa L, Galimand J, Fenneteau O, Mohandas N. Hereditary spherocytosis, elliptocytosis, and other red cell membrane disorders. Blood Reviews. 2013;**27**(4):167-178

[121] White C, Reine N. Feline nonregenerative anaemia: Pathophysiology and etiologies. Compendium of Continuing Education for Veterinarians. 2009;**31**(7):1-7

[122] Li H, Lu L, Li X, Buffet PA, Dao M, Karniadakis GE, et al. Mechanics of diseased red blood cells in human spleen and consequences for hereditary blood disorders. PNAS. 2018;**38**:9574-9579

[123] Sidbury JB, Cornblath M, Fisher J, House E. Glycogen in erythrocytes of patients with glycogen storage disease. Pediatrics. 1961;**27**:103-111

[124] McCullough J. RBCs as targets of infection. Hematology. American Society of Hematology. Education Program. 2014;**1**:404-409

[125] Gallagher PG. Disorders of erythrocyte hydration. Blood. 2017;**130**(25):2699-2108

[126] Ozatli D, Koksal AS, Haznedroglu IC, Simsek H, Karakus S, Buyukasik Y, et al. Erythrocytes: Anemias in chronic liver disease. Hematology (Amsterdam, Netherlands). 2000;**51**:69-76

[127] Kaibara M, Shinozaki T, Kita R, Iwata H, Ujiie H, Sasaki K, Li JY, Sawasaki T, Ogawa H. Analysis of coagulation of blood in different animal species with special reference to procoagulant activity of red blood cell. Journal of Japanese Society of Biochemistry. 2006;**20**(1):35-43

[128] Cavanaugh C, Perazella MA. Urine sediment examination in the diagnosis and management of kidney disease: Core curriculum. American Journal of Kidney Diseases. 2019;**73**(2):258-272

[129] Carelli-Alinovi C, Misiti F. Erythrocytes as potential link between diabetes and Alzheimer's disease. Frontiers in Aging Neuroscience. 2017;**9**:276

[130] Tomaiholo G. Biomechanical properties of red blood cells in health and disease towards microfluidics. Biomicrofludics. 2014;**8**:1-19

[131] Ertan NZ, Bozfukloglu S, Ugurei E, Sonan M, Talcin O. Alterations of erythrocytes rheology and cellular susceptibility in end stage renal disease: Effects of peritoneal dialysis. Plosone. 2017;**12**(2):1-13

[132] Yang DH, Chen CH, Wei CC, Cheng YW. Expression of complements receptor type 1 on erythrocytes in autoimmune diseases. Journal of Molecular Biomarkers and Diagnosis. 2014;**5**(2):1-6

[133] De Rotte MCFJ, den Boer E, de Jong PHP, Phijm SMF, Calasan MB, Weel AE, et al. Methotrexate polyglutamates in erythrocytes are associated with lower disease activity in patients with rheumatoid arthritis. Cupus BMJ. Annal of Rheumatoid Disease. 2015;**74**(2):408-414

[134] Madubueze CC, Chukwu COO, Anyanwu C. Blood transfusion practice in orthopaedics and trauma patients at the Ebonyi State University Teaching Hospital. Orient Journal of Medicine. 2008;**20**(1–4):23-28

[135] Schrijvers D. Management of anemia in cancer patients: Transfusions. The Oncologist. 2011;**16**(3):12-18

[136] Saganuwan SA. Ethnoveterinary values of Nigerian medicinal plants: An overview. European Journal of Medicinal Plants. 2017;**18**(4):1-35

[137] Saganuwan SA, Abdul MS. The prevalence of malaria and its therapeutic implication: A case study of Katcha community. African Journal of Pharmacy and Pharmacology. 2015; **10**(110):212-215

[138] Feldmann H, Geisbert TW. Ebola hemorrhagic fever. Seminar. 2011;**377**: 849-852

[139] Christian JA, Wang J, Kiyatkina N. How old are densed red blood cells? The dog's tale. Blood. 1998;**92**(7):2590-2604

Section 2

Future Perspectives

Chapter 8

The Biology and Therapeutic Applications of Red Blood Cell Extracellular Vesicles

Daniel Xin Zhang, Theodoros Kiomourtzis, Chun Kuen Lam and Minh T.N. Le

Abstract

This chapter focuses on the biology of red blood cell extracellular vesicles (RBCEVs) in normal and diseased conditions, and the potential application of RBCEVs in treatment. Extracellular vesicles (EVs) refer to membranous vesicles secreted by cells into the extracellular environment. EV biology belongs to a rapidly developing field in biomedical sciences. EVs represent a natural mode of cell-to-cell communication, which makes them suitable for delivery of therapeutic agents, such as nucleic acids and proteins, in the body. In particular, RBCEVs feature a wide range of benefits in drug delivery as compared to extracellular vesicles derived from other cell types. In comparison to other delivery systems currently available, RBCEVs are nontoxic, low immunogenic, conveniently obtainable, and easy to use and store. Therefore, RBCEVs boast promising and exceptional advantages in overcoming various limitations of conventional therapeutics.

Keywords: extracellular vesicles, red blood cells, therapy, drug delivery

1. Introduction

In the last decade, we observed a massive upsurge of studies in the field of extracellular vesicles (EVs) [1]. As it is known now, EVs can be loaded with different therapeutic molecules and transport them to recipient cells with little interrogation by the immune system. This property of EVs prompts new possibilities for treatment in various clinical settings [2–4]. In this chapter, we review the biology of EVs as a universal cellular component from a broader perspective, and afterward provide an updated view on red blood cell extracellular vesicles (RBCEVs), their merits and potential applications in therapeutics [5].

2. Overview of extracellular vesicles

2.1 History of extracellular vesicles

Wolf was the first to discover small procoagulant structures derived from activated platelets in human blood and named them "platelet dust" in 1967. He separated the small structures by ultracentrifugation and further characterized them using an electron microscopy [6]. In 1987, Johnstone further studied the formation of such vesicles in the duration of sheep reticulocytes maturation *in vitro*. He was able to identify more activities and characteristics of the vesicles. However, he did not name the small vesicles or discover how they were generated in detail [7]. Both of these findings were important milestones in the field, which allowed for further studies on the function of these small vesicles. Today, we call these small vesicles as EVs. Valadi and colleagues were the first who discovered the natural delivery of microRNAs and mRNAs in EVs in mast cells. Later on, nucleic acid transport via EVs was also observed in many other cell types as an essential manner of intercellular communication [8–10]. We now have a much more profound understanding in the field of EVs due to the continuous efforts of various scientists throughout many decades.

2.2 Biogenesis and compositions of extracellular vesicles

EVs are a heterogeneous class of cell-derived structures with a lipid bilayer membrane, which comprise exosomes, microvesicles, and apoptotic bodies. They are either of the endosomal origins or are shed from the plasma membrane under physiological and pathological conditions. Additionally, they are present in almost all biological fluids, such as blood, urine, breast milk, cerebrospinal fluid, saliva, semen, etc. [11–17]. Further characterizations are based on the different sizes and biogenesis of EVs. Exosomes generally range from 50 to 150 nm in diameter and are secreted from endosomal multivesicular bodies, whereas microvesicles are larger vesicles ranging from 100 to 500 nm in diameter and are formed through a budding or exocytosis process of the plasma membrane [11, 18–23]. Apoptotic bodies are much larger, ranging from 800 to 5000 nm in diameter, and are generated by blebbing of plasma membrane from cells undergoing apoptosis. Hence, apoptotic bodies represent the fragments of dying cells and differ from exosomes and microvesicles in property (**Figure 1**) [17–22]. In this chapter, we will collectively term both exosomes and microvesicles as EVs with apoptotic bodies excluded.

The components of EVs are mainly proteins, lipids, and nucleic acids. However, due to different biogenesis mechanisms, the compositions of exosomes and microvesicles do vary slightly [11, 24–26]. Proteins that are associated with endocytic pathways can be usually found in EVs, such as flotillin and annexin. Some of the biogenesis-associated proteins, such as Tsg101 and Alix, and common tetraspanins, such as CD9 and CD81, are commonly used as EVs markers with CD63 which is mostly regarded as a marker of exosomes. However, currently, there lack well-defined protein markers to distinguish exosomes and microvesicles [11, 24–26]. Lipid components of EVs include phosphatidylcholine, phosphatidylserine, phosphatidylethanolamine, sphingomyelin, cholesterol, and so on, which can be found in plasma membrane as well. As microvesicles are formed by budding from plasma membrame, the lipid composition of microvesicles resembles that of plasma membrane of the cells more while exosomes are of higher levels in sphingomyelin, cholesterol, and phosphatidylserine [27–29]. It is noteworthy that many nucleic acid species are highly enriched in EVs. The lipid bilayer structure of EVs acts as a natural shelter against degrading nucleases in the extracellular environment and protects the nucleic acid cargo under adverse conditions such as long-term storage and multiple freeze-thaw cycles. In the recent decade, reports have it that many mRNAs, microRNAs, and other non-coding RNAs are discovered in EVs (**Figure 1**) [30–32].

2.3 Intercellular communication mediated by extracellular vesicles

As EVs are abundant and widely distributed in biological fluids and carry bioactive cargo, they influence various biological processes of the donor and recipient

DOI: http://dx.doi.org/10.5772/intechopen.81758

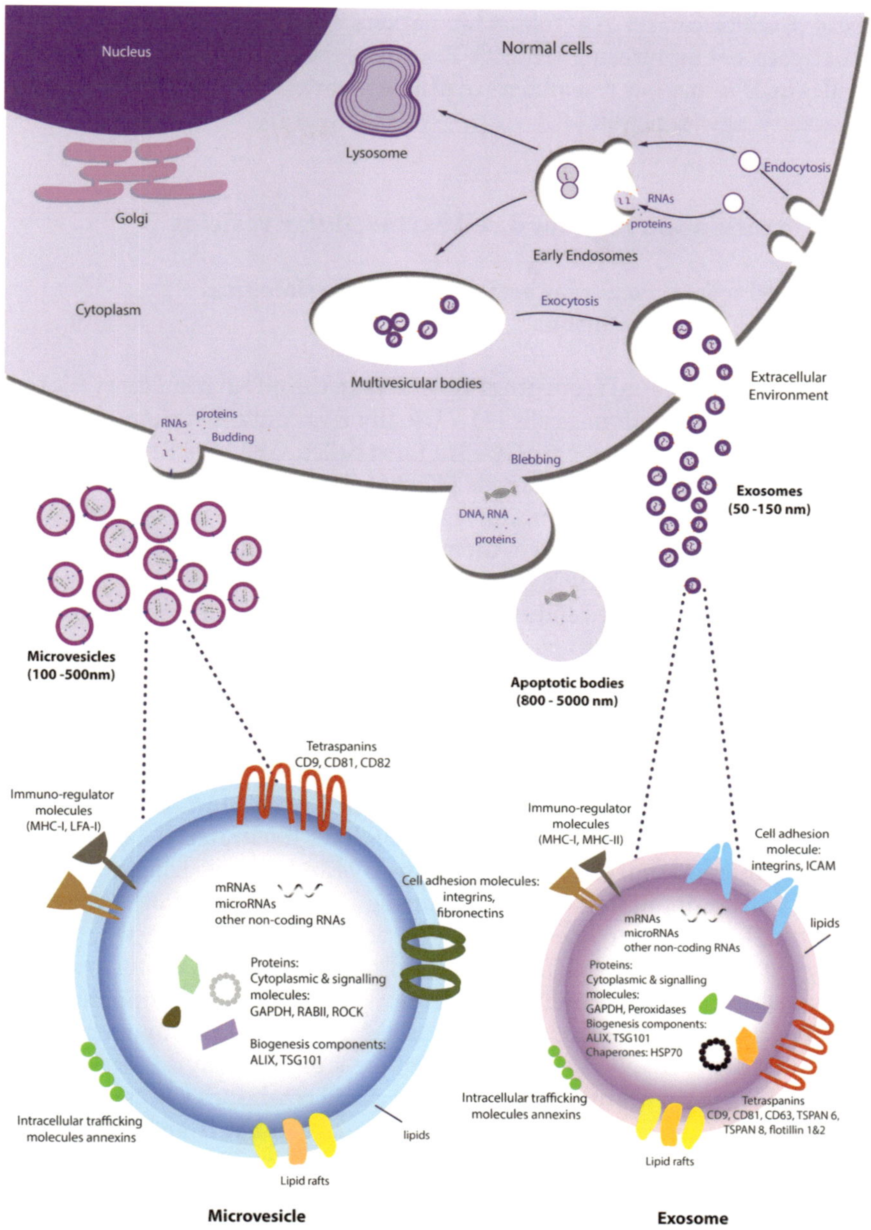

Figure 1.
Biogenesis and composition of extracellular vesicles. Extracellular vesicles (EVs) are composed of exosomes, microvesicles, and apoptotic bodies. Exosomes are typically of endosomal origins and are the smallest among them with 50 to 150 nm in diameter. Microvesicles are larger in size from 100 to 500 nm in diameter and are generated through an outward budding or exocytosis of the plasma membrane. Apoptotic bodies are usually the largest ranging from 800 to 5,000 nm in diameter and are generated by blebbing of plasma membrane from cells undergoing apoptosis. Major components of EVs are lipids, proteins, and nucleic acids. Due to different biogenesis mechanisms, the compositions of exosomes and microvesicles do vary.

cells [33]. The intercellular communication can occur between cells by transferring EVs that act as an exchange mediator of proteins, lipids, and RNAs. Thus, EVs have a fundamental role to play in important biological processes such as the exchange of surface membrane and horizontal RNA transport between neighboring and remote cells [18]. This aspect is being extensively investigated in cancers [34], neurodegenerative diseases [35], autoimmune disorders [36], aging [37], and so on. The bioactive cargo encapsulated by EVs contain valuable information from the source of diseases, which can serve as robust biomarkers in diagnostics and status snapshots in treatment monitoring [38, 39]. The endogenous property of transporting molecules by EVs inspires researchers to utilize them as a superb delivery platform of therapeutic agents as well [40].

3. Concentrations on red blood cell extracellular vesicles

3.1 Red blood cell extracellular vesicles under physiological and pathological conditions

Similar to EVs released from other cells, EVs in the circulation carry biomarkers originated from the donor cells [41]. Usually EVs contain various markers which indicate their origins, e.g., CD235a (also called GPA) for RBCs, CD41 for platelets, and CD11c for dendritic cells [42–44]. RBCs express classes of CD59 and DAF, known as complement inhibitors, and signaling of CD47 and SHPS-1 molecules on the cell surface to protect themselves against endogenous elimination [45, 46]. For instance, the RBCs membrane protein CD47 inhibits RBCs phagocytosis via macrophages by binding to the inhibitory receptor signal regulatory protein alpha (SIRPα). The presence of such proteins on the surfaces of RBCEVs may help RBCEVs to escape from the clearance by macrophages if they carry CD47 on their surfaces [47–49]. Mature RBCs lack nuclei and most of the intracellular membrane structures; hence, EVs released from mature RBCs are microvesicles derived from the plasma membrane (**Figure 2**). Even with the same cell origins, the protein or lipid compositions of EVs may differ on account of the lateral cell membrane variation. Further proteomic assays have illustrated that to some extent, the proteomic spectrum difference of EVs and the releasing cells can be attributed to the stimulating conditions during EVs biogenesis [50]. Microvesicles derived from RBCs are reported to be different in protein contents when produced naturally *in vivo*, *ex vivo* released during cold storage of RBCs, or *in vitro* by treatment with EVs' release-inducing chemicals such as calcium ionophore, even though they seem homogeneous merely based on their size and/or surface markers. The most distinctively different proteins are stomatin and flotillin-2 [51].

There are many studies of RBCEVs under diseased conditions with malaria being frequently reported. Mantel and colleagues illustrated that EVs from human RBCs infected with *Plasmodium falciparum* parasites contain microRNAs that are able to moderate target genes in recipient cells [52]. The infected RBC-derived EVs in malaria were internalized by endothelial cells and the EVs-encapsulated miRNA-Argonaute 2 complexes repressed miRNA target genes and changed endothelial barrier properties. Furthermore, multiple miRNA species in such EVs were identified [52]. Ankarklev and colleagues reviewed the role of RBCEVs in malaria and found that the development of EVs by *Plasmodium* sp. is associated with clinical outcomes [53]. Studies have pointed out that elevated EVs levels were detected in patients with severe malaria cases, and increased EV excretion to the endothelium has been linked to infected RBCs [53].

3.2 Red blood cell extracellular vesicles for therapeutic purposes

Chang and colleagues demonstrated the ability of RBCEVs to efficiently deliver ultra-small superparamagnetic iron oxide particles into human bone marrow mesenchymal stem cells for cellular magnetic resonance imaging *in vitro* and *in vivo* in order to develop successful stem cell therapies [54]. The novel method overcomes the difficulty of relatively low intracellular labeling efficiency and addresses biosafety issues associated in comparison with traditional approaches. RBCEVs were

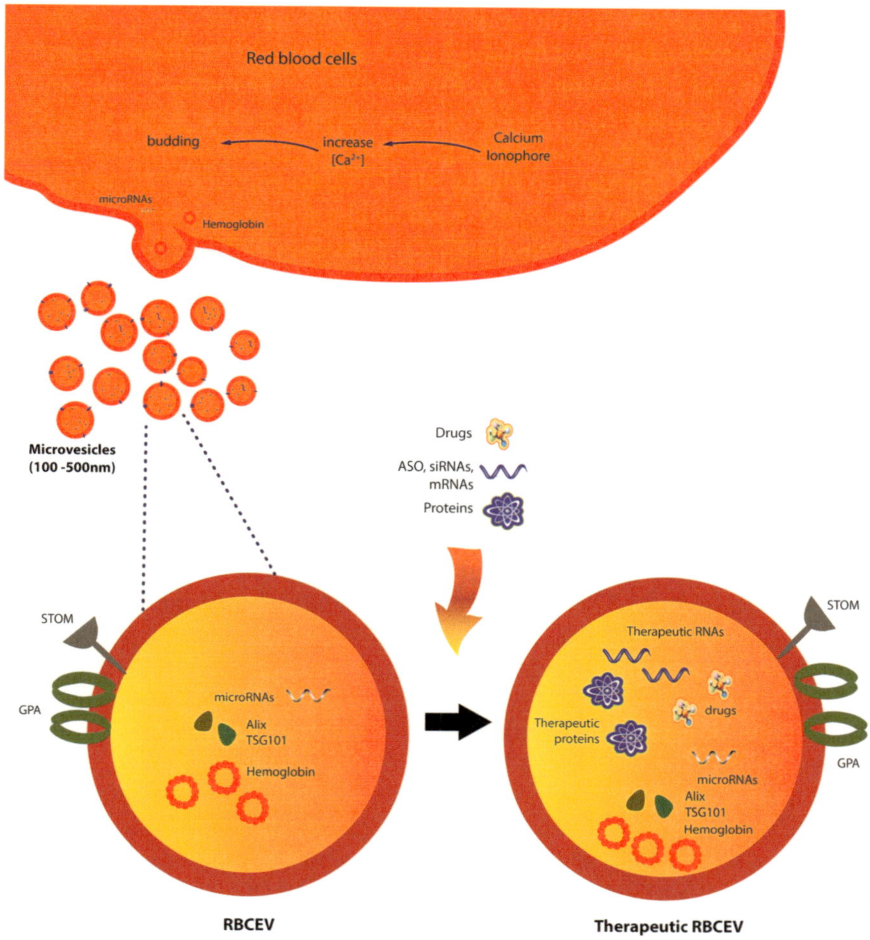

Figure 2.
Using red blood cell extracellular vesicles (RBCEVs) for therapeutic delivery. Calcium ionophore is added to RBCs which simulates the release of microvesicles, the only type of RBCEVs. Naturally, RBCEVs contain hemoglobin, Alix, TSG101, and some microRNAs in their lumen. They also display stomatin (STOM) and glycophorin A (GPA) on their membrane. RBCEVs can be loaded with therapeutic molecules including RNAs, proteins, and chemical drugs for delivery of these molecules to other cell types.

shown to be ultra biosafe and can be used as potential delivery vehicles for clinical applications due to their autologous property to human bone marrow mesenchymal stem cells [54]. Usman and colleagues developed a robust delivery system for RNA-based therapeutics using RBCEVs [55]. Using the novel RBCEVs delivery platform, both small RNA, e.g., antisense oligonucleotides (ASOs), and large RNA, such as Cas9 mRNA, can be electroporated into RBCEVs and transported to target cells in both solid and liquid tumors. In the study, microRNA-125b-ASO-loaded RBCEVs significantly dampened breast tumor growth by intratumoral injection and suppressed acute myeloid leukemia (AML) progression by systemic administration. Genome editing effects were also observed when RBCEVs were loaded with Cas9 mRNA with guide RNAs. The delivery efficiency was higher and far less cytotoxicity was observed as compared to other commercial transfection reagents [55].

3.3 Isolation and loading of red blood cell extracellular vesicles for therapeutic purposes

Up to now, standardized protocols for EVs isolation for either scientific research or clinical application are lacking [56]. One of the commonly used methods to obtain EVs is ultrafiltration with subsequent differential ultracentrifugation. Ultrafiltration followed by liquid size exclusion chromatography suits the large-scale demand of isolating EV for therapeutics as the method results in, on the one hand, a significantly higher EV yield and, on the other hand, the well-preserved biophysical properties of the purified EVs [57]. Usman and colleagues provided a lab-based approach to purify RBCEVs using ultracentrifugation with sucrose cushion. To begin with, RBCs in whole blood were separated from white blood cells and plasma by low centrifugation and using leukodepletion filters. Then, the isolated RBCs were diluted in PBS and treated with 10 mM calcium ionophore overnight which can stimulate the release of RBCEVs and significantly increase the yield. In order to purify RBCEVs, RBCs and cell debris were removed by several rounds of low-speed centrifugation. Later, the resulting supernatants were passed through 0.45 μm syringe filters. Afterward, the RBCEVs were concentrated using ultracentrifugation at 100,000 × *g* for 70 min. Subsequently, RBCEVs were resuspended in cold PBS and layered above frozen 60% sucrose cushion and centrifuged at 100,000 × *g* for 16 h. The red layer of RBCEVs above the sucrose was collected and washed again with cold PBS by ultracentrifugation [55]. The approach is cost-effective, features high RBCEVs yield, and can be adopted in most laboratory settings. The use of sucrose cushion is also a highlight as it helps remove the protein contaminants outside RBCEVs, which might trigger unnecessary immune response and protects the integrity and biophysical properties of RBCEVs.

For therapeutic agents to be loaded into EVs, two major strategies currently have been applied. The first option is to load the therapeutic molecules, such as RNAs, into the EVs after EVs isolation, while the second one is conducted during EV biogenesis. These methods are also known as post-loading and pre-loading, respectively. The pre-loading encapsulation approach is also referred to as the endogenous method as it uses the cellular machinery in order to load small RNA into EVs. The pre-loading approach has been shown to work for the packaging of both siRNA and miRNA into EVs. The post-loading method artificially introduces RNAs into EVs, whereas pre-loading is performed in the EVs biogenesis. Post-loading can be subdivided into passive loading, such as by physical incubation, and active loading with instances of electroporation or sonication. Furthermore, the functional small RNAs delivery using electroporated EVs has been shown to be a success in several reports but it depends on the small RNA species [58–62]. Usman and colleagues used the electroporation method for post-loading of RNAs into RBCEVs [55]. Ideally, various therapeutic molecules including ASOs, siRNAs, gRNAs, mRNAs, plasmid DNA, proteins, peptides, and chemical drug compounds can be loaded into RBCEVs using electroporation (**Figure 2**). Other post-loading methods such as mild sonication and physical incubation may be applicable to RBCEVs as tested for other types of EVs. Labeling of EVs is then required to examine the efficiency of delivery to target cells. Various methods and techniques have been applied to label EVs, with most common methods being incubation with biotinylated radioisotope, substrate of luciferase, fluorescence lipophilic dye, streptavidin-conjugated fluorescence dyes, or the use of other modified proteins [55, 64–66].

3.4 Advantages of red blood cell extracellular vesicles in therapeutics

Due to their innate function on cell-cell communication, EVs can be used effectively for drug delivery [12, 67–69]. The biggest advantage of EVs drug delivery is probably that EVs can be taken from an organism and returned to the same organism *in vivo* after being loaded with therapeutic agents, which are thought to be nonimmunogenic. Another advantage to deliver nucleic acids with the help of EVs is that EVs can carry molecules through physiological barriers, such as the blood-brain barrier, which are hard to cross using conventional delivery methods. Normally, when exogenous RNAs are introduced into the body directly, they will be cleared before reaching the target tissues or cells of interest through degradation by nucleases, or they will be filtered in the kidneys. Both coding and noncoding RNAs were shown to be transferred by EVs intercellular crosstalks. Additionally, it has been shown that microRNAs can be transported in EVs to various cell types. Thus, EVs can be used as a promising vehicle for delivery of RNA-based drugs. Potential fields for therapeutic use include gene therapy, targeted therapy, vaccination, improvement of pregnancy outcome, newborn medicine, kidney disease, and treatment of autoimmune disease [12, 67–69].

It has been reported that diversified types of cells, including RBCs, endothelial cells, monocytes, granulocytes, and platelets, release EVs. Additionally, EVs can be isolated by various methods from cell culture media, plasma, and other biofluids [23, 41, 70, 71]. Although several research groups have demonstrated the advantages of using EVs for RNA delivery, there are still issues with EVs generated from fibroblasts and dendritic cells being not permanently available from all subjects [69, 72]. RBCs are readily obtainable from any human subject and easy to store, and blood transfusion has been a relatively safe, well-established, and routine medical procedure for decades which makes RBCEVs easy to obtain and safe to use. Thus, EVs from whole plasma are easily accessible and substantially present, but these EVs are derived from various cell types, e.g., nucleated cells which represent a risk for horizontal gene transfer [63]. Therefore, obtaining ultrapure RBCEVs solely derived from RBCs is highly preferred as RBCs lack both nuclear and mitochondrial DNA, which means that RBCEVs for pharmaceutical purpose avoid the risk of horizontal gene transfer. RBCEVs formation has been extensively investigated and described in the recent years. Therefore, with such knowledge, RBCEVs are safer and less complicated to use [73–76].

Consequently, RBCEVs possess several features which make them better suitable for clinical applications than EVs from other cell types. First of all, blood units are easily accessible from existing blood banks. A large scale of RBCEVs can be produced at low cost as RBCs are the most abundant cell type in the body (84% of all cells) and, during their 120-day lifespan, RBCs continue to release RBCEVs, leading to an approximate 20% loss in RBCs volume and an increase of around 14% in hemoglobin concentration [23, 77–79]. Additionally, RBCEVs are obtainable for allogeneic and autologous transfusion from the patients' own blood. A large number of RBCs (~10^{12} cells/L) are obtainable from each blood unit. Thus, there exists no need to expand cells in culture and no risk of the emergence of mutations *in vitro*. In addition, no cGMP-qualified media or supplements are required, which are financially desirable. Large-scale amounts (10^{13}–10^{14}) of RBCEVs can be isolated from RBCs (per unit) when treated with calcium ionophore, which is a scalable strategy to obtain EVs. Secondly, RBCEVs are safer compared to EVs from other cell types, because the enucleated RBCs contain no DNA, unlike EVs from nucleated cell types which represent a potential risk for horizontal gene transfer. As plasma EVs are heterogeneous with unpredictable contents, RBCEVs are safer than plasma EVs for allogeneic treatments of cancer because cancer cells and immune cells are known to release large amounts of cancer-promoting EVs into their environment [80, 81]. Thirdly, RBCEVs are nontoxic; hence, they are safer as compared to the toxic synthetic transfection reagents which are typically used. As mentioned before, RNAs in RBCEVs are stable and completely functional *in vitro* and in *vivo* for both liquid and solid cancers. Fourthly, RBCEVs are presumably nonimmunogenic via blood type matching, unlike adenoviruses, adeno-associated viruses, lentiviruses, nanoparticles, and various synthetic transfection reagents. Last but not least, RBCEVs can be frozen and thawed many cycles without affecting their integrity or efficacy. This fact suggests that RBCEVS can be developed into stable pharmaceutical products in the future, but further research needs to be done. Compared to most other current methods for programmable RNA drug therapies, which are unsuitable for the clinical use because of the low uptake efficiency and high cytotoxicity, RBCEVs show promising future prospects [55].

4. Conclusion

EVs are shed from the plasma membrane or released by endosomal pathways under both physiological and diseased conditions. Intercellular communication is one of the best known functions of EVs by far, which provides the possibility to utilize the EVs natural vehicle property of transporting nucleic acids, proteins, and lipids for drug delivery. Recent studies demonstrate that human RBCEVs can be developed as robust delivery platform for multiple therapeutic RNAs in cancer treatment. RBCEVs feature multiple benefits as compared to EVs from other cell types. They are easily obtainable in large amounts, can be frozen and thawed multiple times without significant compromise, are nontoxic and nonimmunogenic, can reach remote tissues in the body with minimal hindrance by physiological barriers, and do not contain DNA or other unpredictable contents which could result in horizontal gene transfer. By obtaining RBCEVs directly from the patient, they are safe to use allogeneic treatments and possess no risk of emerging mutations during expansion by cell culture. Thus, RBCEVs show promising advantages in overcoming various limitations of cell-based therapeutics. All in all, RBCEVs need further research in order to establish them as a new source and promising approach for practical therapeutics in clinical use.

Acknowledgements

We would like to thank our colleagues at City University of Hong Kong including Chin Siew Mei, Waqas Muhammad Usman, Tin Chanh Pham, Luyen Tien Vu, Boya Peng, Thach Tuan Pham, Abdullah Faqeer, Yeokyeong Kim, Seongkyeol Kim, Likun Wei, Ching Yee Moo, Ru Zhen, and Migara Kavishka Jayasinghe for their support. We are grateful to the generous funding from the Hong Kong Health, and Medical Research Fund (grant 03141186) and the Hong Kong Research Grants Council (grant 21106616).

Conflict of interest

The authors declare no conflict of interest.

Author details

Daniel Xin Zhang[1†], Theodoros Kiomourtzis[2†], Chun Kuen Lam[1] and Minh T.N. Le[1,3]*

1 Department of Biomedical Sciences, Jockey Club College of Veterinary Medicine and Life Sciences, City University of Hong Kong, Kowloon, Hong Kong

2 Eberhard Karls University of Tübingen, Tübingen, Germany

3 City University of Hong Kong Shenzhen Research Institute, Shenzhen, P.R. China

*Address all correspondence to: mle.bms@cityu.edu.hk

† These authors contributed equally.

References

[1] Roy S, Hochberg FH, Jones PS. Extracellular vesicles: The growth as diagnostics and therapeutics: A survey. Journal of Extracellular Vesicles. 2018;**7**(1):1438720. PubMed PMID: 29511461. Pubmed Central PMCID: 5827771

[2] Masaoutis C, Mihailidou C, Tsourouflis G, Theocharis S. Exosomes in lung cancer diagnosis and treatment. From the translating research into future clinical practice. Biochimie. 2018;**151**:27-36. PubMed PMID: 29857182

[3] Pan J, Ding M, Xu K, Yang C, Mao LJ. Exosomes in diagnosis and therapy of prostate cancer. Oncotarget. 2017;**8**(57):97693-97700. PubMed PMID: 29228644. Pubmed Central PMCID: 5722596

[4] Li A, Zhang T, Zheng M, Liu Y, Chen Z. Exosomal proteins as potential markers of tumor diagnosis. Journal of Hematology and Oncology. 2017;**10**(1):175. PubMed PMID: 29282096. Pubmed Central PMCID: 5745959

[5] Gyorgy B, Hung ME, Breakefield XO, Leonard JN. Therapeutic applications of extracellular vesicles: Clinical promise and open questions. Annual Review of Pharmacology and Toxicology. 2015;**55**:439-464. PubMed PMID: 25292428. Pubmed Central PMCID: 4445965

[6] Wolf P. The nature and significance of platelet products in human plasma. British Journal of Haematology. 1967;**13**(3):269-288. PubMed PMID: 6025241

[7] Johnstone RM, Adam M, Hammond JR, Orr L, Turbide C. Vesicle formation during reticulocyte maturation. Association of plasma membrane activities with released vesicles (exosomes). The Journal of Biological Chemistry. 1987;**262**(19):9412-9420. PubMed PMID: 3597417

[8] Valadi H, Ekstrom K, Bossios A, Sjostrand M, Lee JJ, Lotvall JO. Exosome-mediated transfer of mRNAs and microRNAs is a novel mechanism of genetic exchange between cells. Nature Cell Biology. 2007;**9**(6):654-659. PubMed PMID: 17486113

[9] Kosaka N, Yoshioka Y, Hagiwara K, Tominaga N, Katsuda T, Ochiya T. Trash or treasure: Extracellular microRNAs and cell-to-cell communication. Frontiers in Genetics. 2013;**4**:173. PubMed PMID: 24046777. Pubmed Central PMCID: 3763217

[10] Vader P, Breakefield XO, Wood MJ. Extracellular vesicles: Emerging targets for cancer therapy. Trends in Molecular Medicine. 2014;**20**(7):385-393. PubMed PMID: 24703619. Pubmed Central PMCID: 4082760

[11] van Niel G, D'Angelo G, Raposo G. Shedding light on the cell biology of extracellular vesicles. Nature Reviews Molecular Cell Biology. 2018;**19**(4):213-228. PubMed PMID: 29339798

[12] Lee Y, El Andaloussi S, Wood MJ. Exosomes and microvesicles: Extracellular vesicles for genetic information transfer and gene therapy. Human Molecular Genetics. 2012;**21**(R1):R125-R134. PubMed PMID: 22872698

[13] Nair S, Tang KD, Kenny L, Punyadeera C. Salivary exosomes as potential biomarkers in cancer. Oral Oncology. 2018;**84**:31-40. PubMed PMID: 30115473

[14] Welch JL, Kaddour H, Schlievert PM, Stapleton JT, Okeoma CM. Semen exosomes promote transcriptional

silencing of HIV-1 by disrupting NF-kB/Sp1/Tat circuitry. Journal of Virology. 2018;**92**(21):e00731-18. PubMed PMID: 30111566

[15] Chen CY, Hogan MC, Ward CJ. Purification of exosome-like vesicles from urine. Methods in Enzymology. 2013;**524**:225-241. PubMed PMID: 23498743. Pubmed Central PMCID: 4028690

[16] Martin C, Patel M, Williams S, Arora H, Sims B. Human breast milk-derived exosomes attenuate cell death in intestinal epithelial cells. Innate Immunity. 2018;**24**(5):278-284. PubMed PMID: 29991305

[17] Anderson MR, Pleet ML, Enose-Akahata Y, Erickson J, Monaco MC, Akpamagbo Y, et al. Viral antigens detectable in CSF exosomes from patients with retrovirus associated neurologic disease: Functional role of exosomes. Clinical and Translational Medicine. 2018;**7**(1):24. PubMed PMID: 30146667. Pubmed Central PMCID: 6110307

[18] Kanada M, Bachmann MH, Hardy JW, Frimannson DO, Bronsart L, Wang A, et al. Differential fates of biomolecules delivered to target cells via extracellular vesicles. Proceedings of the National Academy of Sciences of the United States of America. 2015;**112**(12):E1433-E1442. PubMed PMID: 25713383. Pubmed Central PMCID: 4378439

[19] Inal JM, Kosgodage U, Azam S, Stratton D, Antwi-Baffour S, Lange S. Blood/plasma secretome and microvesicles. Biochimica et Biophysica Acta. 2013;**1834**(11):2317-2325. PubMed PMID: 23590876

[20] Nguyen DB, Ly TB, Wesseling MC, Hittinger M, Torge A, Devitt A, et al. Characterization of microvesicles released from human red blood cells. Cellular Physiology and Biochemistry: International Journal of Experimental Cellular Physiology, Biochemistry, and Pharmacology. 2016;**38**(3):1085-1099. PubMed PMID: 26938586

[21] Foller M, Huber SM, Lang F. Erythrocyte programmed cell death. IUBMB Life. 2008;**60**(10):661-668. PubMed PMID: 18720418

[22] Lang F, Gulbins E, Lerche H, Huber SM, Kempe DS, Foller M. Eryptosis, a window to systemic disease. Cellular Physiology and Biochemistry: International Journal of Experimental Cellular Physiology, Biochemistry, and Pharmacology. 2008;**22**(5-6):373-380. PubMed PMID: 19088418

[23] Zmigrodzka M, Guzera M, Miskiewicz A, Jagielski D, Winnicka A. The biology of extracellular vesicles with focus on platelet microparticles and their role in cancer development and progression. Tumour Biology : The Journal of the International Society for Oncodevelopmental Biology and Medicine. 2016;**37**(11):14391-14401. PubMed PMID: 27629289. Pubmed Central PMCID: 5126185

[24] Zaborowski MP, Balaj L, Breakefield XO, Lai CP. Extracellular vesicles: Composition, biological relevance, and methods of study. Bioscience. 2015;**65**(8):783-797. PubMed PMID: 26955082. Pubmed Central PMCID: 4776721

[25] Sinha A, Principe S, Alfaro J, Ignatchenko A, Ignatchenko V, Kislinger T. Proteomic profiling of secreted proteins, exosomes, and microvesicles in cell culture conditioned media. Methods in Molecular Biology. 1722;**2018**:91-102. PubMed PMID: 29264800

[26] Rosa-Fernandes L, Rocha VB, Carregari VC, Urbani A, Palmisano G. A perspective on extracellular vesicles proteomics. Frontiers in Chemistry. 2017;**5**:102. PubMed PMID: 29209607. Pubmed Central PMCID: 5702361

[27] Record M, Silvente-Poirot S, Poirot M, Wakelam MJO. Extracellular vesicles: Lipids as key components of their biogenesis and functions. Journal of Lipid Research. 2018;**59**(8):1316-1324. PubMed PMID: 29764923. Pubmed Central PMCID: 6071772

[28] Pollet H, Conrard L, Cloos AS, Tyteca D. Plasma membrane lipid domains as platforms for vesicle biogenesis and shedding? Biomolecules. 2018;**14**:8(3). PubMed PMID: 30223513

[29] Llorente A, Skotland T, Sylvanne T, Kauhanen D, Rog T, Orlowski A, et al. Molecular lipidomics of exosomes released by PC-3 prostate cancer cells. Biochimica et Biophysica Acta. 2013;**1831**(7):1302-1309. PubMed PMID: 24046871

[30] Momen-Heravi F, Getting SJ, Moschos SA. Extracellular vesicles and their nucleic acids for biomarker discovery. Pharmacology and Therapeutics. 2018;**3**. PubMed PMID: 30081050

[31] Quesenberry PJ, Aliotta J, Deregibus MC, Camussi G. Role of extracellular RNA-carrying vesicles in cell differentiation and reprogramming. Stem Cell Research and Therapy. 2015;**6**:153. PubMed PMID: 26334526. Pubmed Central PMCID: 4558901

[32] Sun L, Meckes DG Jr. Methodological approaches to study extracellular vesicle miRNAs in Epstein-Barr virus-associated cancers. International Journal of Molecular Sciences. 2018;**19**(9):2810. PubMed PMID: 30231493

[33] Yanez-Mo M, Siljander PR, Andreu Z, Zavec AB, Borras FE, Buzas EI, et al. Biological properties of extracellular vesicles and their physiological functions. Journal of Extracellular Vesicles. 2015;**4**:27066. PubMed PMID: 25979354. Pubmed Central PMCID: 4433489

[34] Minciacchi VR, Freeman MR, Di Vizio D. Extracellular vesicles in cancer: Exosomes, microvesicles and the emerging role of large oncosomes. Seminars in Cell and Developmental Biology. 2015;**40**:41-51. PubMed PMID: 25721812. Pubmed Central PMCID: 4747631

[35] Izadpanah M, Seddigh A, Ebrahimi Barough S, Fazeli SAS, Ai J. Potential of extracellular vesicles in neurodegenerative diseases: Diagnostic and therapeutic indications. Journal of Molecular Neuroscience. 2018;**66**(2):172-179. PubMed PMID: 30140997

[36] Fu H, Hu D, Zhang L, Tang P. Role of extracellular vesicles in rheumatoid arthritis. Molecular Immunology. 2018;**93**:125-132. PubMed PMID: 29175592

[37] Robbins PD. Extracellular vesicles and aging. Stem Cell Investigation. 2017;**4**:98. PubMed PMID: 29359137. Pubmed Central PMCID: 5762993

[38] Muinelo-Romay L, Casas-Arozamena C, Abal M. Liquid biopsy in endometrial cancer: New opportunities for personalized oncology. International Journal of Molecular Sciences. 2018;**19**(8):2311. PubMed PMID: 30087246. Pubmed Central PMCID: 6121388

[39] Samandari M, Julia MG, Rice A, Chronopoulos A, Del Rio Hernandez AE. Liquid biopsies for management of pancreatic cancer. Translational Research : The Journal of Laboratory and Clinical Medicine. 2018;**201**:98-127. PubMed PMID: 30118658

[40] Jiang L, Vader P, Schiffelers RM. Extracellular vesicles for nucleic acid delivery: Progress and prospects for safe RNA-based gene therapy. Gene Therapy. 2017;**24**(3):157-166. PubMed PMID: 28140387

[41] Wu YW, Goubran H, Seghatchian J, Burnouf T. Smart blood cell and microvesicle-based Trojan horse drug delivery: Merging expertise in blood transfusion and biomedical engineering in the field of nanomedicine. Transfusion and Apheresis Science : Official Journal of the World Apheresis Association : Official Journal of the European Society for Haemapheresis. 2016;**54**(2):309-318. PubMed PMID: 27179926

[42] Chung SM, Bae ON, Lim KM, Noh JY, Lee MY, Jung YS, et al. Lysophosphatidic acid induces thrombogenic activity through phosphatidylserine exposure and procoagulant microvesicle generation in human erythrocytes. Arteriosclerosis, Thrombosis, and Vascular Biology. 2007;**27**(2):414-421. PubMed PMID: 17110600

[43] Kina T, Ikuta K, Takayama E, Wada K, Majumdar AS, Weissman IL, et al. The monoclonal antibody TER-119 recognizes a molecule associated with glycophorin A and specifically marks the late stages of murine erythroid lineage. British Journal of Haematology. 2000;**109**(2):280-287. PubMed PMID: 10848813

[44] Burnier L, Fontana P, Kwak BR, Angelillo-Scherrer A. Cell-derived microparticles in haemostasis and vascular medicine. Thrombosis and Haemostasis. 2009;**101**(3):439-451. PubMed PMID: 19277403

[45] Oldenborg PA, Zheleznyak A, Fang YF, Lagenaur CF, Gresham HD, Lindberg FP. Role of CD47 as a marker of self on red blood cells. Science. 2000;**288**(5473):2051-2054. PubMed PMID: 10856220

[46] Ishikawa-Sekigami T, Kaneko Y, Okazawa H, Tomizawa T, Okajo J, Saito Y, et al. SHPS-1 promotes the survival of circulating erythrocytes through inhibition of phagocytosis by splenic macrophages. Blood. 2006;**107**(1):341-348. PubMed PMID: 16141346

[47] Burger P, Hilarius-Stokman P, de Korte D, van den Berg TK, van Bruggen R. CD47 functions as a molecular switch for erythrocyte phagocytosis. Blood. 2012;**119**(23):5512-5521. PubMed PMID: 22427202

[48] Burger P, de Korte D, van den Berg TK, van Bruggen R. CD47 in erythrocyte ageing and clearance—The Dutch point of view. Transfusion Medicine and Hemotherapy : Offizielles Organ der Deutschen Gesellschaft fur Transfusionsmedizin und Immunhamatologie. 2012;**39**(5):348-352. PubMed PMID: 23801927. Pubmed Central PMCID: 3678269

[49] Per-Arne O. Role of CD47 and signal regulatory protein alpha (SIRPalpha) in regulating the clearance of viable or aged blood cells. Transfusion Medicine and Hemotherapy : Offizielles Organ der Deutschen Gesellschaft fur Transfusionsmedizin und Immunhamatologie. 2012;**39**(5):315-320. PubMed PMID: 23801922. Pubmed Central PMCID: 3678265

[50] Ratajczak J, Wysoczynski M, Hayek F, Janowska-Wieczorek A, Ratajczak MZ. Membrane-derived microvesicles: Important and underappreciated mediators of cell-to-cell communication. Leukemia. 2006;**20**(9):1487-1495. PubMed PMID: 16791265

[51] Prudent M, Crettaz D, Delobel J, Seghatchian J, Tissot JD, Lion N. Differences between calcium-stimulated and storage-induced erythrocyte-derived microvesicles. Transfusion and Apheresis Science: Official Journal of the World Apheresis Association: Official Journal of the European Society for Haemapheresis. 2015;**53**(2):153-158. PubMed PMID: 26549671

[52] Mantel PY, Hjelmqvist D, Walch M, Kharoubi-Hess S, Nilsson S, Ravel D, et al. Infected erythrocyte-derived extracellular vesicles alter vascular function via regulatory Ago2-miRNA complexes in malaria. Nature Communications. 2016;**7**:12727. PubMed PMID: 27721445. Pubmed Central PMCID: 5062468

[53] Ankarklev J, Hjelmqvist D, Mantel PY. Uncovering the role of erythrocyte-derived extracellular vesicles in malaria: From immune regulation to cell communication. Journal of Circulating Biomarkers. 2014;**3**:3

[54] Chang M, Hsiao JK, Yao M, Chien LY, Hsu SC, Ko BS, et al. Homologous RBC-derived vesicles as ultrasmall carriers of iron oxide for magnetic resonance imaging of stem cells. Nanotechnology. 2010;**21**(23):235103. PubMed PMID: 20479509

[55] Usman WM, Pham TC, Kwok YY, Vu LT, Ma V, Peng B, et al. Efficient RNA drug delivery using red blood cell extracellular vesicles. Nature Communications. 2018;**9**(1):2359. PubMed PMID: 29907766. Pubmed Central PMCID: 6004015

[56] Lotvall J, Hill AF, Hochberg F, Buzas EI, Di Vizio D, Gardiner C, et al. Minimal experimental requirements for definition of extracellular vesicles and their functions: A position statement from the International Society for extracellular vesicles. Journal of Extracellular Vesicles. 2014;**3**:26913. PubMed PMID: 25536934. Pubmed Central PMCID: 4275645

[57] Nordin JZ, Lee Y, Vader P, Mager I, Johansson HJ, Heusermann W, et al. Ultrafiltration with size-exclusion liquid chromatography for high yield isolation of extracellular vesicles preserving intact biophysical and functional properties. Nanomedicine : Nanotechnology, Biology, and Medicine. 2015;**11**(4):879-883. PubMed PMID: 25659648

[58] Didiot MC, Haraszti RA, Aronin N, Khvorova A. Loading of extracellular vesicles with hydrophobically modified siRNAs. Methods in Molecular Biology. 1740;**2018**:199-214. PubMed PMID: 29388146

[59] Haraszti RA, Coles A, Aronin N, Khvorova A, Didiot MC. Loading of extracellular vesicles with chemically stabilized hydrophobic siRNAs for the treatment of disease in the central nervous system. Bio-Protocol. 2017;**20**:7(20). PubMed PMID: 28868334. Pubmed Central PMCID: 5580947

[60] Vader P, Kooijmans SA, Stremersch S, Raemdonck K. New considerations in the preparation of nucleic acid-loaded extracellular vesicles. Therapeutic Delivery. 2014;**5**(2):105-107. PubMed PMID: 24483187

[61] Johnsen KB, Gudbergsson JM, Skov MN, Pilgaard L, Moos T, Duroux M. A comprehensive overview of exosomes as drug delivery vehicles—Endogenous nanocarriers for targeted cancer therapy. Biochimica et Biophysica Acta. 2014;**1846**(1):75-87. PubMed PMID: 24747178

[62] van der Meel R, Fens MH, Vader P, van Solinge WW, Eniola-Adefeso O, Schiffelers RM. Extracellular vesicles as drug delivery systems: Lessons from the liposome field. Journal of Controlled Release : Official Journal of the Controlled Release Society. 2014;**195**: 72-85. PubMed PMID: 25094032

[63] Wahlgren J, De LKT, Brisslert M, Vaziri Sani F, Telemo E, Sunnerhagen P, et al. Plasma exosomes can deliver exogenous short interfering RNA to monocytes and lymphocytes. Nucleic Acids Research. 2012;**40**(17):e130. PubMed PMID: 22618874. Pubmed Central PMCID: 3458529

[64] Lamichhane TN, Jeyaram A, Patel DB, Parajuli B, Livingston NK,

Arumugasaamy N, et al. Oncogene knockdown via active loading of small RNAs into extracellular vesicles by sonication. Cellular and Molecular Bioengineering. 2016;**9**(3):315-324. PubMed PMID: 27800035. Pubmed Central PMCID: 5084850

[65] Lamichhane TN, Raiker RS, Jay SM. Exogenous DNA loading into extracellular vesicles via electroporation is size-dependent and enables limited gene delivery. Molecular Pharmaceutics. 2015;**12**(10):3650-3657. PubMed PMID: 26376343. Pubmed Central PMCID: 4826735

[66] Kotmakci M, Bozok CV. Extracellular vesicles as natural nanosized delivery systems for small-molecule drugs and genetic material: Steps towards the future nanomedicines. Journal of Pharmacy and Pharmaceutical Sciences : A Publication of the Canadian Society for Pharmaceutical Sciences, Societe Canadienne des Sciences Pharmaceutiques. 2015;**18**(3):396-413. PubMed PMID: 26517135

[67] Lv LL, Wu WJ, Feng Y, Li ZL, Tang TT, Liu BC. Therapeutic application of extracellular vesicles in kidney disease: Promises and challenges. Journal of Cellular and Molecular Medicine. 2018;**22**(2):728-737. PubMed PMID: 29083099. Pubmed Central PMCID: 5783839

[68] Willis GR, Kourembanas S, Mitsialis SA. Therapeutic applications of extracellular vesicles: Perspectives from newborn medicine. Methods in Molecular Biology. 1660;**2017**:409-432. PubMed PMID: 28828676

[69] Kamerkar S, LeBleu VS, Sugimoto H, Yang S, Ruivo CF, Melo SA, et al. Exosomes facilitate therapeutic targeting of oncogenic KRAS in pancreatic cancer. Nature. 2017;**546**(7659):498-503. PubMed PMID: 28607485. Pubmed Central PMCID: 5538883

[70] Alchinova IB, Khaspekova SG, Golubeva NV, Shustova ON, Antonova OA, Karganov MY, et al. Comparison of the size of membrane microparticles of different cellular origin by dynamic light scattering. Doklady Biochemistry and Biophysics. 2016;**470**(1):322-325

[71] Wu ZH, Ji CL, Li H, Qiu GX, Gao CJ, Weng XS. Membrane microparticles and diseases. European Review for Medical and Pharmacological Sciences. 2013;**17**(18):2420-2427. PubMed PMID: 24089218

[72] Alvarez-Erviti L, Seow Y, Yin H, Betts C, Lakhal S, Wood MJ. Delivery of siRNA to the mouse brain by systemic injection of targeted exosomes. Nature Biotechnology. 2011;**29**(4):341-345. PubMed PMID: 21423189

[73] Bevers EM, Comfurius P, Dekkers DW, Zwaal RF. Lipid translocation across the plasma membrane of mammalian cells. Biochimica et Biophysica Acta. 1999;**1439**(3):317-330. PubMed PMID: 10446420

[74] Daleke DL. Regulation of transbilayer plasma membrane phospholipid asymmetry. Journal of Lipid Research. 2003;**44**(2):233-242. PubMed PMID: 12576505

[75] Gonzalez LJ, Gibbons E, Bailey RW, Fairbourn J, Nguyen T, Smith SK, et al. The influence of membrane physical properties on microvesicle release in human erythrocytes. PMC Biophysics. 2009;**2**(1):7. PubMed PMID: 19703298. Pubmed Central PMCID: 2739839

[76] Bevers EM, Williamson PL. Phospholipid scramblase: An update. FEBS Letters. 2010;**584**(13):2724-2730. PubMed PMID: 20302864

[77] Shi J, Kundrat L, Pishesha N, Bilate A, Theile C, Maruyama T, et al. Engineered red blood cells as carriers for systemic delivery of a wide array of functional probes. Proceedings of

the National Academy of Sciences of the United States of America. 2014;**111**(28):10131-10136. PubMed PMID: 24982154. Pubmed Central PMCID: 4104923

[78] Sender R, Fuchs S, Milo R. Revised estimates for the number of human and bacteria cells in the body. PLoS Biology. 2016;**14**(8):e1002533. PubMed PMID: 27541692. Pubmed Central PMCID: 4991899

[79] Bosman GJ, Werre JM, Willekens FL, Novotny VM. Erythrocyte ageing in vivo and in vitro: Structural aspects and implications for transfusion. Transfusion Medicine. 2008;**18**(6): 335-347. PubMed PMID: 19140816

[80] Kalluri R. The biology and function of exosomes in cancer. The Journal of Clinical Investigation. 2016;**126**(4):1208-1215. PubMed PMID: 27035812. Pubmed Central PMCID: 4811149

[81] Kosaka N, Yoshioka Y, Fujita Y, Ochiya T. Versatile roles of extracellular vesicles in cancer. The Journal of Clinical Investigation. 2016;**126**(4):1163-1172. PubMed PMID: 26974161. Pubmed Central PMCID: 4811151

Chapter 9

Application of Red Cell Membrane in Nanobiotechnology

Insu Kim, Gyudo Lee and Dae Sung Yoon

Abstract

Red cells are full of unique biological properties such as immune evasion and molecular-specific permeability. These properties originate from various membrane proteins on the surface of the cell membrane. For this reason, red cell membrane is coated on nanomaterials or sensors to bestow the functionalities of the membrane proteins. In this chapter, various types of membrane proteins of red cell and its functions are described. Also, the following two experimental procedures are summarized: (I) the extraction of red cell membrane containing membrane proteins and (II) coating of the extracted cell membrane onto the nanoparticles and solid surface of sensors. Finally, the applications of red cell membrane in drug delivery system and biosensor are discussed.

Keywords: red cell membrane, membrane proteins, cell membrane coating, biosensors

1. Introduction

Red cells (RCs), also called as erythrocyte, are the most abundant cells in the body and highly specialized in gas transportation [1]. RCs deliver oxygen from the lungs to all body tissues and carry carbon dioxide to the lungs. For the delivery of the gases, RCs circulate through blood vessels to the whole body without being trapped inside narrow capillary vessels (5–10 μm in diameter) which are smaller than the size of RCs [2]. Also, RCs do not get attacked by immune system such as mononuclear phagocytic system (MPS) and complement system (CS) [3, 4]. The unique characteristics of the RCs come from specialized microstructure of RC. The microstructure of RC has a biconcave disc-like shape and is fully packed with hemoglobin instead of nucleus and intracellular organelles. Also, various membrane proteins and carbohydrates are embedded in the cell membrane which characterizes intrinsic functionalities of RCs [5]. The biconcave disc-like shape maximizes the surface area of the cell, which increases the gas exchanges between internal and external gases. Hemoglobins are oxygen-transport metalloproteins that bind gases such as oxygen and carbon dioxide. Especially, membrane proteins of RC are responsible for numerous characteristics such as permeability to specific molecules (e.g., glucose, urea, and gases), immune evasive properties, unique biconcave disc-like structure, flexibility, and deformability [4, 6]. Recently, it is reported that membrane proteins of RC can be utilized by manipulating the cell membrane [7]. The RC membrane (RCM) inside the whole blood of mice or human contains membrane proteins, which were extracted and purified. Accordingly, intriguing researches were conducted together. For example, just like RC does, RCM-coated nanoparticles showed long circulation in the blood by evading immune responses such as MPS and CS [7, 8]. Also, RCM-coated glucose sensors showed high perm-selectivity to glucose [9]. As a result, the sensor was barely affected by interfering molecules such as saccharides and antioxidants. Likewise, the utilization of the functionalities of membrane protein of RC advances nanobiotechnology in the field of drug delivery system and biosensor. In this chapter, we investigate the various membrane proteins expressed on RC and its functionalities. The techniques for extraction and functionalization of cell membrane have been researched. Also, we discuss about the application of RCM functionalization for the last decade.

2. Membrane proteins of red cell membrane and its functionalities

Membrane proteins are essential components allowing specific functionalities for cells. There are three categories classified by its function. Membrane proteins perform as receptors, transporters, and cell adhesion molecules. **Table 1** represents major membrane proteins on RCM classified by their function [5].

2.1 Membrane receptors

Membrane receptors are one of integral membrane proteins. They mediate cell signaling via binding extracellular molecules. Specifically, membrane receptors allow communication between the cell and external environment. Hormones, cytokines, cell adhesion molecules, and immunoproteins are examples of the extracellular molecules. The ligand bound of the membrane receptor may induce changes in the metabolism or activity of the cell. In RC, CD55 (decay-accelerating factor) and

Protein	Gene	Function
Membrane receptor		
CD55 ([a]DAF)	CD55	Decay-accelerating factor that prevents the activation of complement system
CD59	CD59	[b]MAC-inhibitory protein that prevents complement membrane attack complex
Transporter		
AE1 (band 3)	SLC4A1	Anion transporter
RhAG	RhAG	Ammonia transporter
Nucleoside transporter	SLC29A1	Nucleoside transporter
Urea transporter	SLC14A1	Urea transporter
Glucose transporter	SLC2A	Glucose transporter
Cell adhesion molecule		
CD47	CD47	"do not eat me" signal protein that interacts with [c]SIRPα to inhibit phagocytosis

Membrane receptors consist of CD55 and CD59; transporters consist of AE1, RhAG, nucleoside transporter, urea transporter, and glucose transporter; cell adhesion molecule consists of CD47.
[a]DAF, decay-accelerating factor.
[b]MAC, membrane attack complex.
[c]SIRPα, signal regulatory protein alpha.

Table 1.
Various membrane proteins in RCs [5].

CD59 are well-known membrane receptors which inhibit CS preventing hemolysis (**Figure 1**) [10]. In detail, CS is composed of proximal and terminal complement (**Figure 2**) [4]. The proximal CS has three pathways converged at the step of complement component 3 (C3) activation. The terminal complement is initiated with complement component 5 (C5) and ended with formation of membrane attack complex (MAC). In this cascade, CD55 inhibits C3 activation by deactivating C3 convertase [11]. CD59 inhibits terminal complement activation by preventing the formation of MAC that starts with the activation of C5 [12]. The absence of CD55 and CD59 may lead to hemolysis of RC via complement activation [4].

2.2 Transporters

Transporters are involved in the movement of specific molecules or ions across cell membrane. The proteins are involved in the movement of molecules by active transport or facilitated diffusion. It is revealed that anion, gas, nucleoside, urea, and glucose transporters are expressed on the RC. In detail, (AE1, also called band 3) is responsible for mediating the exchange of chloride ion with bicarbonate (HCO_3^-) across RCM [13]. Rh-associated glycoprotein (RhAG) is a gas transporter which permeates carbon dioxide [1]. Nucleoside transporter mediates the transport of nucleoside substrates like adenosine [14]. Urea transporter is specialized in urea transportation, which is activated by antidiuretic hormone (vasopressin) [15]. Glucose transporter (GLUT) is a uniporter that transports glucose toward intracellular orientation (**Figure 3**) [16]. GLUT is an essential protein for glucose uptake of the cell by catalyzing facilitative diffusion. Especially, RC expresses a large number of GLUT compared to other cells because the cell lacks mitochondria and the energy is produced by glycolysis of glucose [17].

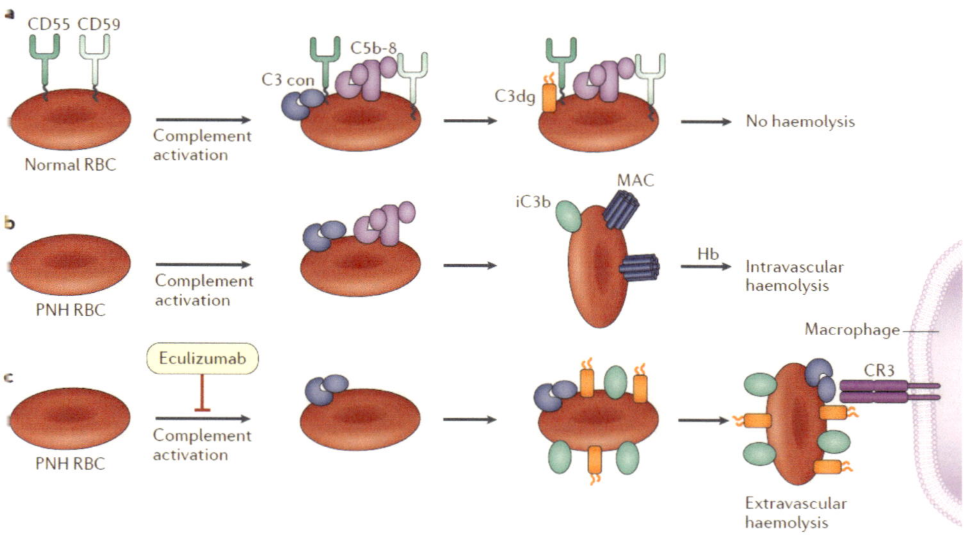

Figure 1.
*Hemolysis mechanism of paroxysmal nocturnal hemoglobinuria (PNH) via the complement system [4]. (a) Normal RBC possesses CD55 and CD59 which are glycosylphosphatidylinositol (GPI)-anchored self-protective complement regulatory factors. CD55 is a widely expressed membrane protein that accelerates the decay of C3 convertases. CD59 is the major inhibitor of terminal complement, which blocks the generation of the membrane attack complex (MAC). (b) Intravascular hemolysis of PNH RBC through C3 convertase and MAC. (c) Extravascular hemolysis of PNH RBC via macrophage. Eculizumab inhibits the complement activation by compensating CD59. *PNH, a life-threatening disease characterized by destruction of RBC by complement system; eculizumab, a monoclonal antibody complement inhibitor which is highly effective for PNH; C3 con, C3 convertase; C5b-8, complex of C5b, C6, C7, and C8 proteins; C3dg, a fragment of C3 protein, which is ligand of integrin (CR3) on macrophage; iC3b, inactivated C3b; Hb, hemoglobin; CR3, complementary 3.*

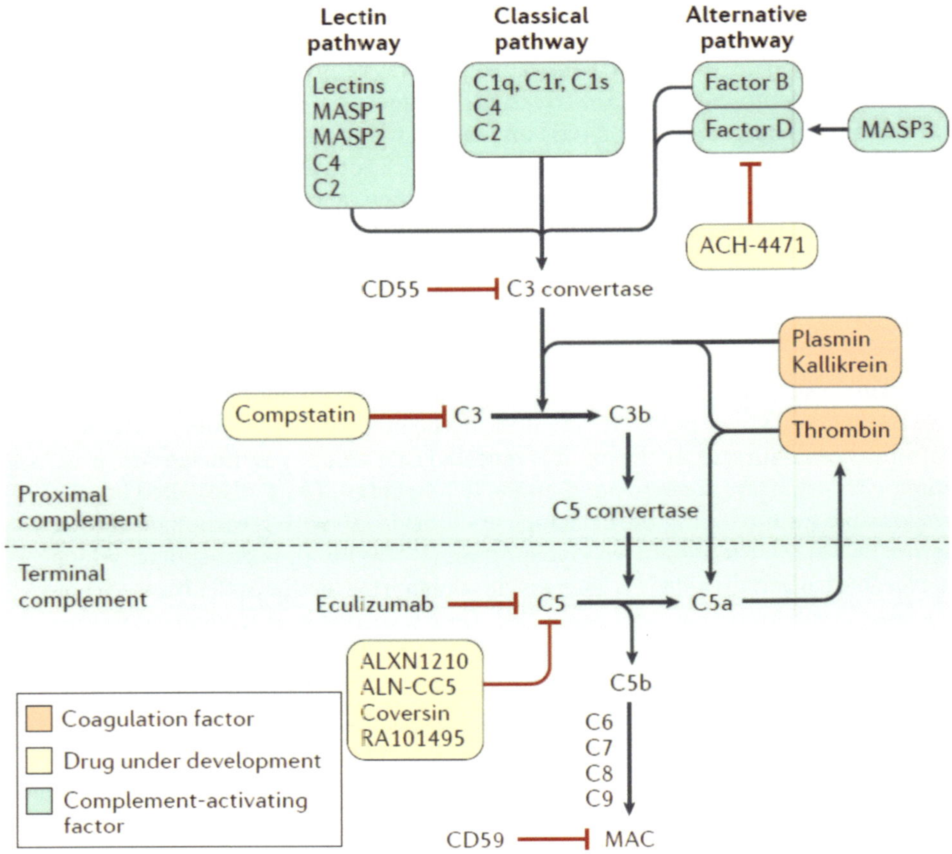

Figure 2.
Complement system signal cascade [4]. Proximal complement consists of three pathways. The lectin, classical, and alternative pathways initiate and converge at the step of complement component 3 (C3) activation. Terminal complement is initiated by C5 convertases, leading to cleavage of C5 to C5a and C5b. C5b oligomerizes with C6, C7, C8, and multiple C9 molecules to form the membrane attack complex (MAC). The CD55 inhibits proximal complement activation by accelerating the decay of C3 convertases preventing the incorporation of C9 into the MAC.

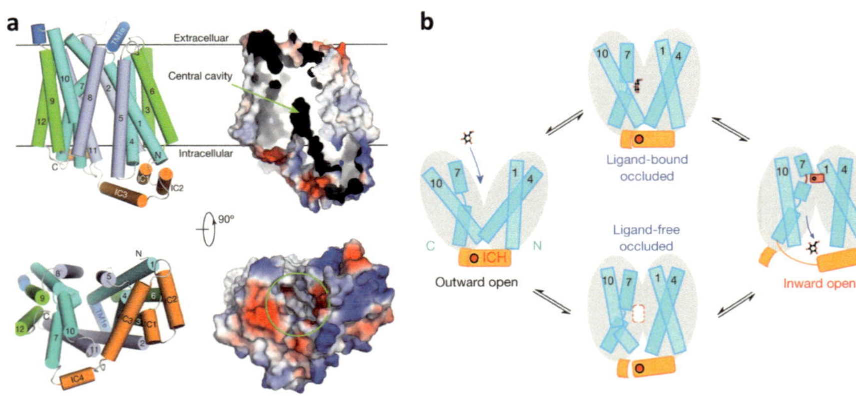

Figure 3.
(a) Overall structure of human glucose transporter-1 (GLUT1) and (b) working model for GLUT1 [16]. The working model is predicted to have four conformations (outward open, ligand-bound and occluded, inward-open, and ligand-free and occluded) required for a complete glucose transport cycle. Intracellular helix (ICH) domain of GLUT1 has two critical roles. First, the ICH domain appears to maintain a defined conformation with respect to the N domain. Second, the ICH domain is pulled toward the C domain during the inter-domain rotation from occluded to inward-open conformation.

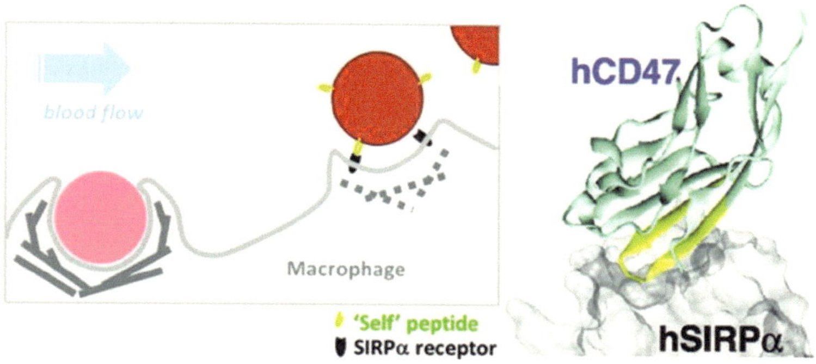

Figure 4.
The cocrystal structure shows human CD47 (hCD47) with human signal regulatory protein α (hSIRPα). The left panel depicts that the occurrence of phagocytosis depends on the reaction between hCD47 and hSIRPα [6].

2.3 Cell adhesion molecules

Cell adhesion molecules interact with membrane receptors of various cells. RC has CD47 as a cell adhesion molecule [18]. CD47 belongs to the immunoglobulin superfamily and sends a "*don't eat me*" signal to MPS such as monocyte and macrophage (**Figure 4**) [6]. This intriguing signal is derived from the interaction between CD47 and signal regulatory protein alpha (SIRPα) which is expressed on monocytes and most of subpopulations such as macrophages. Indeed, CD47-eliminated RCs were easily phagocytosed by macrophages unlike RC with CD47 [3, 19].

3. Red cell membrane extraction and functionalization techniques

3.1 Red cell membrane extraction procedure

RC can easily be extracted from whole blood of mice or human. Normally, the whole blood is extracted at vacutainer tube (evacuated tube) containing anticoagulant such as heparin, citrate, or ethylenediaminetetraacetic acid (EDTA) according to the purpose (**Table 2**). Heparin collection tubes are preferred for peripheral blood in cytogenic studies. Heparin activates antithrombin III which deactivates thrombin and serine endopeptidase, which are essential enzymes for coagulation [20]. Citrate collection tubes are employed for blood transfusion and coagulation assays because citrate reversibly binds to calcium which is an essential molecule in many steps of coagulation cascade [21]. EDTA collection tubes are usually used for complete blood count (CBC) test because EDTA is a strong anticoagulant that irreversibly binds to calcium [22]. Since coagulation requires RC to form blood clot, EDTA collection tubes are mostly used for RC extraction [7, 8, 23].

The procedure for extracting RC from whole blood is as follows [23]. Whole blood withdrawn from mice or human is centrifuged at 800–1000 g for 5 min at 4°C in order to remove the plasma and the buffy coat. The resulting sediment is washed three times with ice-cold 1× PBS to remove blood proteins adsorbed on RCs. To extract cell membrane from RCs, hypotonic treatment, homogenize, or sonication is conducted for hemolysis. Hypotonic treatment is the most convenient hemolysis procedure without disruption of membrane and membrane proteins. Washed RCs are suspended in 0.25× PBS for 20 min at 4°C. As hemolysis progresses, hemoglobin is released from RCs, and RC ghosts (empty cell membrane without cytoplasmic contents) are formed [24]. As a result, RC ghost can be verified with phase contrast

Anticoagulant	Usage	Mechanism
Heparin	Cytogenetic studies	Activate antithrombin III which deactivates serum clotting factors (factors [a]IIa and [b]Xa)
Citrate	Coagulation assays, blood transfusion	Bind to calcium reversibly (not as strong as EDTA)
Ethylenediaminetetraacetic acid (EDTA)	molecular genetic studies, complete blood counts	Strongly bind to calcium irreversibly. The absence of calcium

[a]*Factor IIa, thrombin.*
[b]*factor Xa, serine endopeptidase.*

Table 2.
Vacutainers with various anticoagulants.

microscope. To remove the hemoglobin, hemolyzed solution is centrifuged and washed. Then the RCM is collected with light pink pellet. The resulting RCM concentrate is stored in −70°C before use.

3.2 Red cell membrane coating techniques on nanoparticle and solid surface

Cell membrane coating technology comes from phospholipid manipulation technique which forms liposome and solid-supported lipid bilayer because the phospholipids are the main component of cell membrane. Although the phospholipid manipulation technique was developed quite a while ago, cell membrane coating techniques on nanoparticles were first reported in 2011 (**Figure 5**) [7]. Researchers prepared RCM-coated nanoparticles by RCM vesicle-nanoparticle fusion [25, 26]. Specifically, the extracted cell membrane was adequately diluted (membrane extraction was described in Section 3.1.). For the membrane vesicle derivation, outer forces are applied to the diluted membrane. Sonicating the membrane is the easiest way to make membrane vesicle, but it is hard to regulate the size of the vesicle. Alternatively, extrusion methods can control the size of the membrane vesicle by porous polymer membrane with various pore sizes. Next, membrane coating onto nanoparticles is conducted with the same procedure to

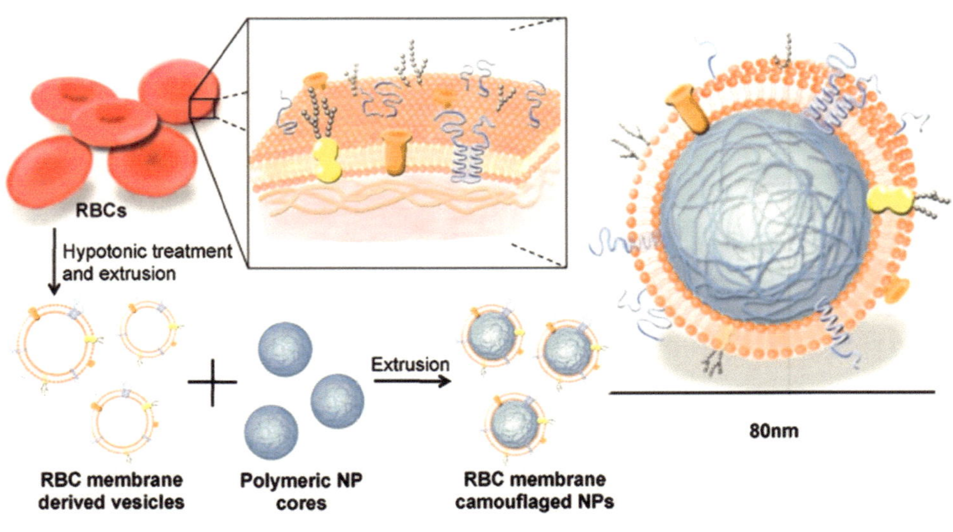

Figure 5.
The schematic illustration of the preparation of RBC membrane-coated polymeric nanoparticles [7]. RBCs, red blood cell; polymeric NP, polymeric nanoparticle such as poly(lactic-co-glycolic acid) (PLGA) nanoparticle.

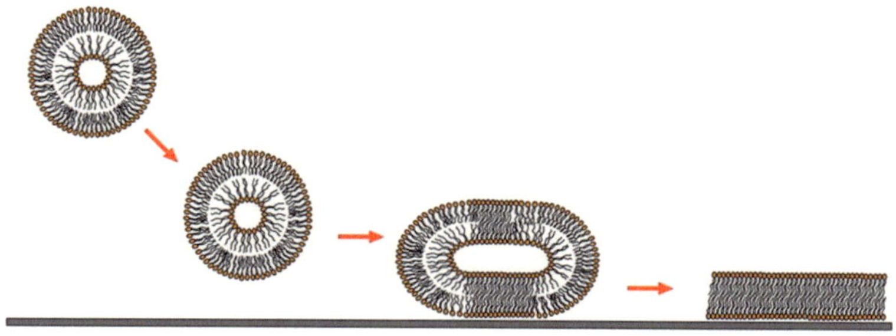

Figure 6.
Fusion of a lipid vesicle on solid surface [27].

vesicle formation (i.e., sonication or extrusion). In detail, the prepared membrane vesicles are mixed with nanoparticles. Then the sonication or extrusion of the mixture can lead to the coating of membrane onto the nanoparticles by the principle of vesicle fusion.

The cell membrane coating on solid surface is similar to that on nanoparticles described above. The coating procedure is based on vesicle fusion method (**Figure 6**) [27]. The only different procedure for solid surface coating is that thermal energy is employed instead of mechanical energy (i.e., sonication or extrusion) [9, 28]. Specifically, the cell membrane vesicles with adequate concentration were placed on solid surface and incubated for 45 min at 50°C. The thermal energy induces the membrane vesicle to collide and fuse onto the solid surface. It is noted that the temperature for vesicle fusion should be lower than the denaturation temperature of proteins to avoid the deactivation or misfolding by high thermal energy [29].

4. The applications of red cell membrane in drug delivery systems and biosensors

RCM-coated nanoparticles, also called RC-camouflaged nanoparticles, have been developed for drug delivery system since they were devised by Zhang and his group in 2011. It was found that immune evasive properties of RCM-coated nanoparticles are superior to conventional nanoparticles. The membrane proteins confer the advantages of the immune avoidance properties described in Section 2. RCM coating has been applied to various core nanoparticles such as gold, poly(lactic-co-glycolic acid) (PLGA), silica, and iron oxide nanoparticles [30]. Also, RCM can be utilized as permselective filter for glucose biosensor taking advantage of GLUT on RCM [9].

4.1 Drug delivery with red cell membrane-coated nanoparticles

In drug delivery system related with nanomaterial, long-term circulation of nanoparticles in vivo is one of the most important characteristics because various immune responses clear the foreign molecules in the body and blood [31]. Especially, MPS and CS are major immune systems eliminating drug delivery carriers. Conventionally, to evade the immune systems, the drug carriers are functionalized with polyethylene glycol (PEG) which slows clearance in blood and avoids non-specific binding of blood proteins [32, 33]. In our body, however, there is an anti-PEG immunological response which removes PEGylated nanoparticles [34]. By contrast, the RCM-coated nanoparticles showed prolonged circulation in blood. The result is exactly attributed to membrane receptors and cell adhesion molecules, which were abundant and diverse on RCM. In this regard, the immune evasive properties of RCM-functionalized nanomaterials have great potential as clinical drug delivery carriers. In particular, it is researched that the RCM-functionalized nanoparticles showed good dispersion stability in serum and great biodistribution in mice model up to 72 h (**Figure 7**) [7]. Indeed, it is demonstrated that the RCM inhibits macrophage uptake. RCM-coated gold nanoparticles showed ~4 times higher immune evasive properties than bare gold nanoparticles [8].

4.2 Permselective glucose sensing with red cell membrane-coated biosensors

In biosensors, not only sensitivity but also specificity (selectivity) is important because numerous molecules coexist in the biological samples that may interfere the detection [35]. For example, blood contains ions, saccharides, proteins, and blood cells which hinder accurate glucose detection. Enzymatic glucose biosensors, most widely used, employ glucose oxidase or glucose dehydrogenase

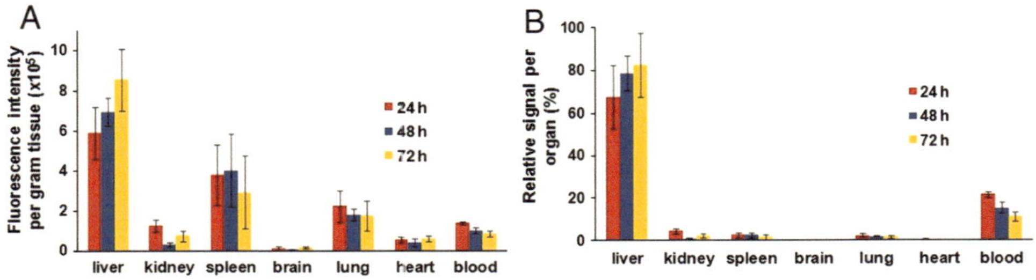

Figure 7.
Biodistribution of RCM-coated gold nanoparticles in mice [7]. The fluorescently labeled nanoparticles were injected intravenously into the mice. The fluorescent intensity at the liver, kidney, spleen, brain, lung, heart, and blood was measured at 24, 48, and 72 h. (A) fluorescent intensity per gram of tissue (n = 6). (B) Relative signal per organ.

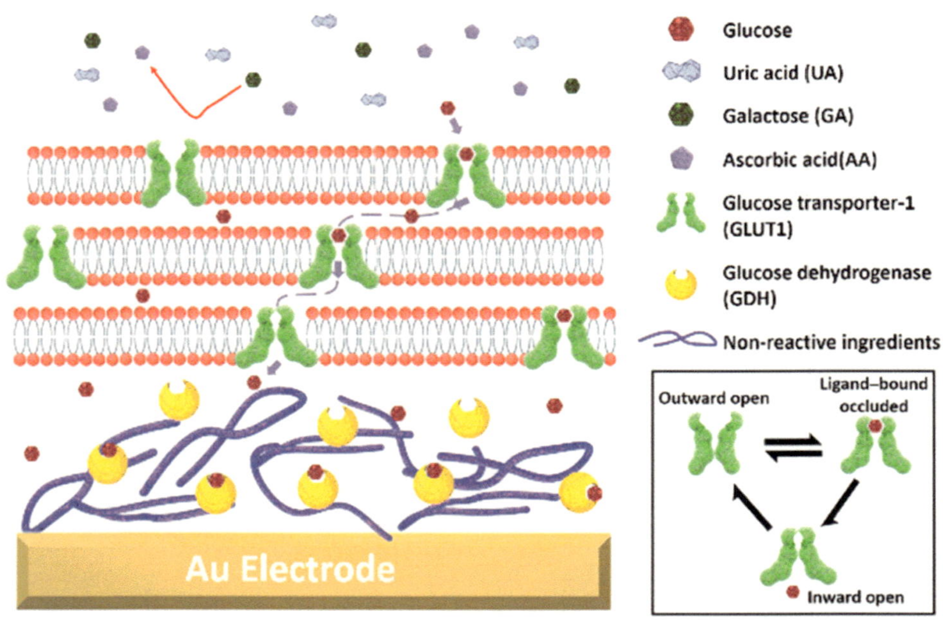

Figure 8.
Schematic illustration of RCM-coated glucose sensor [9]. The RCM-coated enzymatic glucose sensor specifically reacts with glucose via taking advantage of glucose transporter-1 (GLUT1).

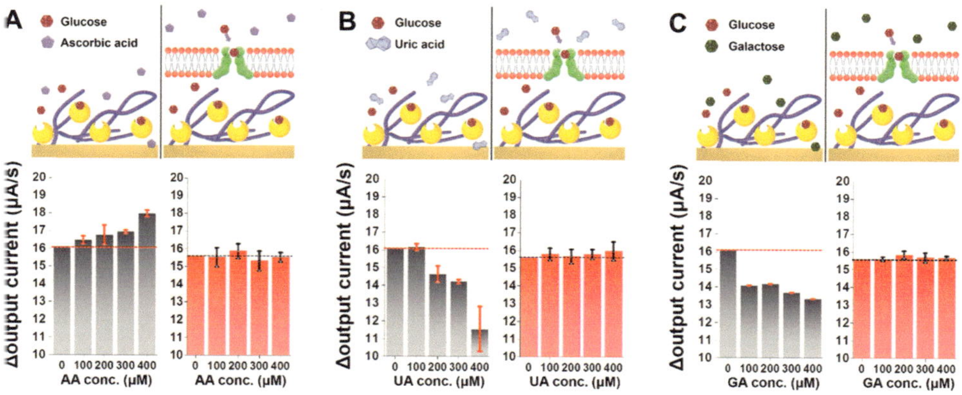

Figure 9.
Selectivity test of RCM-coated glucose sensors under competitive interactions between glucose and each interfering molecule [9]. The selectivity test was conducted with 5 mM of glucose blended with each interfering molecule, e.g. (A) ascorbic acid (AA), (B) uric acid (UA), or (C) galactose (GA). The black and red bars represent the output signal of uncoated sensor and RCM-coated sensor, respectively.

for selective detection of glucose. However, the enzymes react with glucose and other similar structured molecules (mono- and disaccharides) such as fructose, galactose, and maltose in blood. For this reason, glucose sensors are interfered by the molecules. It is reported that RCM which has glucose transporter was employed as glucose-selective permeable membrane by taking advantage of GLUT (**Figure 8**) [9]. The RCM-coated sensor showed high selectivity to glucose compared to uncoated sensor. In detail, the uncoated sensors are highly affected by the increment of interfering molecules (e.g., ascorbic acid, uric acid, and galactose), whereas the RCM-coated sensors exhibit consistency in glucose detection. In particular, RCM-coated sensor showed that the signals of glucose with interfering molecules barely change from that of glucose without interfering molecules (**Figure 9**) [9].

5. Conclusions

The RCM has various types of membrane proteins such as membrane receptor, transporter, and cell adhesion molecules. Each type of membrane proteins is full in potentials to be applied in various fields such as drug delivery system and biosensor. The well-evolved functionality of membrane proteins can be easily utilized by coating the RCM on nanomaterial and solid surface of sensors. Currently, drug delivery system is the major field of RCM application because the membrane can confer the immune evasive properties of RCM to the nanomaterials. In the future, it is expected that the RCM will be increasingly applied in development of highly selective biosensors utilizing various transporters on RCM.

Acknowledgements

This work was supported by the National Research Foundation of Korea (NRF) Grant funded by the Korean Government (MSIP) (No. NRF-2016R1A2B4010269, NRF-2017R1A6A3A11034311 and NRF-2018M3C1B7020722). This material is also supported by the Ministry of Trade, Industry and Energy (MOTIE, Korea) under Industrial Technology Innovation Program (No.10079316). Gyudo Lee is thankful for the financial support by Korea University Grant.

Author details

Insu Kim, Gyudo Lee* and Dae Sung Yoon*
School of Biomedical Engineering, Korea University, Seoul, Korea

*Address all correspondence to: lkd0807@korea.ac.kr and dsyoon@korea.ac.kr

References

[1] Mohandas N, Gallagher PG. Red cell membrane: Past, present, and future. Blood. 2008;**112**(10):3939-3948. DOI: 10.1182/blood-2008-07-161166

[2] Steck TL. The organization of proteins in the human red blood cell membrane. A review. The Journal of Cell Biology. 1974;**62**(1):1-19

[3] Oldenborg P-A et al. Role of CD47 as a marker of self on red blood cells. Science. 2000;**288**(5473):2051-2054. DOI: 10.1126/science.288.5473.2051

[4] Hill A et al. Paroxysmal nocturnal haemoglobinuria. Nature Reviews Disease Primers. 2017;**3**:17028. DOI: 10.1038/nrdp.2017.28

[5] Bryk AH, Wiśniewski JR. Quantitative analysis of human red blood cell proteome. Journal of Proteome Research. 2017;**16**(8):2752-2761. DOI: 10.1021/acs.jproteome.7b00025

[6] Barclay AN, van den Berg TK. The interaction between signal regulatory protein alpha (SIRPα) and CD47: Structure, function, and therapeutic target. Annual Review of Immunology. 2014;**32**(1):25-50. DOI: 10.1146/annurev-immunol-032713-120142

[7] Hu C-MJ et al. Erythrocyte membrane-camouflaged polymeric nanoparticles as a biomimetic delivery platform. Proceedings of the National Academy of Sciences. 2011;**108**(27):10980-10985. DOI: 10.1073/pnas.1106634108

[8] Gao W et al. Surface functionalization of gold nanoparticles with red blood cell membranes. Advanced Materials. 2013;**25**(26):3549-3553. DOI: 10.1002/adma.201300638

[9] Kim I et al. A highly permselective electrochemical glucose sensor using red blood cell membrane. Biosensors and Bioelectronics. 2018;**102**:617-623. DOI: 10.1016/j.bios.2017.12.002

[10] Sugimori C et al. Minor population of CD55-CD59- blood cells predicts response to immunosuppressive therapy and prognosis in patients with aplastic anemia. Blood. 2006;**107**(4):1308-1314. DOI: 10.1182/blood-2005-06-2485

[11] Maillard N et al. Current understanding of the role of complement in IgA nephropathy. Journal of the American Society of Nephrology. 2015;**26**(7):1503-1512. DOI: 10.1681/asn.2014101000

[12] Tegla CA et al. Membrane attack by complement: The assembly and biology of terminal complement complexes. Immunologic Research. 2011;**51**(1):45. DOI: 10.1007/s12026-011-8239-5

[13] Peters LL et al. Anion exchanger 1 (band 3) is required to prevent erythrocyte membrane surface loss but not to form the membrane skeleton. Cell. 1996;**86**(6):917-927. DOI: 10.1016/S0092-8674(00)80167-1

[14] Thorn JA, Jarvis SM. Adenosine transporters. General Pharmacology: The Vascular System. 1996;**27**(4):613-620. DOI: 10.1016/0306-3623(95)02053-5

[15] Timmer RT et al. Localization of the urea transporter UT-B protein in human and rat erythrocytes and tissues. American Journal of Physiology-Cell Physiology. 2001;**281**(4):C1318-C1325. DOI: 10.1152/ajpcell.2001.281.4.C1318

[16] Deng D et al. Crystal structure of the human glucose transporter GLUT1. Nature. 2014;**510**:121. DOI: 10.1038/nature13306

[17] Calesnick B, Altarelli VR, Spirtes MA. Decrease in aerobic glycolysis of erythrocytes following the continuous administration of L-triiodothronine.

Endocrinology. 1960;**66**(4):517-520. DOI: 10.1210/endo-66-4-517

[18] Klei TRL et al. From the cradle to the grave: The role of macrophages in erythropoiesis and erythrophagocytosis. Frontiers in Immunology. 2017;**8**(73): 1-13. DOI: 10.3389/fimmu.2017.00073

[19] Tsai RK, Discher DE. Inhibition of "self" engulfment through deactivation of myosin-II at the phagocytic synapse between human cells. The Journal of Cell Biology. 2008;**180**(5):989. DOI: 10.1083/jcb.200708043

[20] Machovich R. Mechanism of action of heparin through thrombin on blood coagulation. Biochimica et Biophysica Acta (BBA) - Protein Structure. 1975;**412**(1):13-17. DOI: 10.1016/0005-2795(75)90334-7

[21] Calatzis A et al. Citrate anticoagulation for extracorporeal circuits: Effects on whole blood coagulation activation and clot formation. Nephron. 2001;**89**(2):233-236. DOI: 10.1159/000046075

[22] Zucker MB, Borrelli J. Some effects of divalent cations on the clotting mechanism and the platelets of EDTA blood. Journal of Applied Physiology. 1958;**12**(3):453-460. DOI: 10.1152/jappl.1958.12.3.453

[23] Jiang Q et al. Red blood cell membrane-camouflaged melanin nanoparticles for enhanced photothermal therapy. Biomaterials. 2017;**143**:29-45. DOI: 10.1016/j.biomaterials.2017.07.027

[24] Gordesky SE, Marinetti GV, Segel GB. Differences in the reactivity of phospholipids with FDNB in normal RBC, sickle cells and RBC ghosts. Biochemical and Biophysical Research Communications. 1972;**47**(5):1004-1009. DOI: 10.1016/0006-291X(72)90932-1

[25] Escajadillo T et al. A red blood cell membrane-camouflaged nanoparticle counteracts streptolysin O-mediated virulence phenotypes of invasive group A streptococcus. Frontiers in Pharmacology. 2017;**8**(477):1-10. DOI: 10.3389/fphar.2017.00477

[26] Zhang Y et al. Erythrocyte membrane-coated nanogel for combinatorial antivirulence and responsive antimicrobial delivery against Staphylococcus aureus infection. Journal of Controlled Release. 2017;**263**:185-191. DOI: 10.1016/j.jconrel.2017.01.016

[27] Mingeot-Leclercq M-P et al. Atomic force microscopy of supported lipid bilayers. Nature Protocols. 2008;**3**:1654. DOI: 10.1038/nprot.2008.149

[28] Katsaras J, Kučerka N, Nieh M-P. Structure from substrate supported lipid bilayers (review). Biointerphases. 2008;**3**(2):FB55-FB63. DOI: 10.1116/1.2992133

[29] Tanford C. Protein denaturation. Advances in Protein Chemistry. 1968;**23**:121-282. DOI: 10.1016/S0065-3233(08)60241-7

[30] Fang RH et al. Cell membrane coating nanotechnology. Advanced Materials. 2018;**30**(23):1706759. DOI: 10.1002/adma.201706759

[31] Danhier F, Feron O, Préat V. To exploit the tumor microenvironment: Passive and active tumor targeting of nanocarriers for anti-cancer drug delivery. Journal of Controlled Release. 2010;**148**(2):135-146. DOI: 10.1016/j.jconrel.2010.08.027

[32] Guo J et al. Aptamer-functionalized PEG–PLGA nanoparticles for enhanced anti-glioma drug delivery. Biomaterials. 2011;**32**(31):8010-8020. DOI: 10.1016/j.biomaterials.2011.07.004

[33] Wang H et al. Enhanced anti-tumor efficacy by co-delivery of doxorubicin and paclitaxel with amphiphilic methoxy PEG-PLGA copolymer nanoparticles. Biomaterials. 2011;**32**(32):8281-8290. DOI: 10.1016/j.biomaterials.2011.07.032

[34] Ishida T et al. PEGylated liposomes elicit an anti-PEG IgM response in a T cell-independent manner. Journal of Controlled Release. 2007;**122**(3):349-355. DOI: 10.1016/j.jconrel.2007.05.015

[35] Moatti-Sirat D, Velho G, Reach G. Evaluating in vitro and in vivo the interference of ascorbate and acetaminophen on glucose detection by a needle-type glucose sensor. Biosensors and Bioelectronics. 1992;**7**(5):345-352. DOI: 10.1016/0956-5663(92)85030-E

Chapter 10

The Influence of the Golden Ratio on the Erythrocyte

Marcy C. Purnell and Risa D. Ramsey

Abstract

Erythrocytes must maintain a biconcave discoid shape in order to efficiently operate and serve an important physiological role in an organism. The erythrocyte can be viewed as a toroidal dielectrophoretic (DEP) electromagnetic field (EMF)-driven cell that maintains its zeta potential via a dielectric constant (chloride anion) that resides between a negatively charged membrane surface and a positively charged Stern layer. There are ferromagnetic (iron) and ferroelectric (chloride anion) influences that may be crucial to the maintenance of this zeta potential. We hypothesize that within this uniquely shaped cell resides an interesting geometric mathematical measure, the Golden Ratio, that houses a DEP EMF may be driven/fueled by the zeta potential and may be critical for the efficient recycling of CO2 and the delivery of O2 to organisms.

Keywords: erythrocyte, chloride anion, Golden Ratio, dielectrophoretic field

1. Introduction

Erythrocytes have a distinct biconcave discoid shape that is necessary for their efficient delivery of oxygen as well as the recycling of carbon dioxide [1]. The mechanisms that drive and maintain this most abundant cell in the body and its unique shape (geometry) have been poorly defined and understood to date [2]. We hypothesize that the erythrocyte is a small toroidal dielectrophoretic electromagnetic field (DEP EMF)-driven cell that maintains its zeta potential via a dielectric constant (chloride anion) between the negatively charged plasma membrane surface and the positively charged Stern (cation) layer [3, 4].

The zeta potential/DEP EMF is driven by both the ferroelectric influences (chloride anion) and the ferromagnetic influences (iron cation) in order to maintain both the Golden Ratio, which is a function of phi (φ), and/or their signature biconcave discoid shape [3]. Within this unique cell's Golden Ratio resides a DEP electromagnetic field flow fractionation (EMFFF) process that carries out the efficient recycling of carbonic acid ($H_2CO_3^-$) into a proton (H^+) that participates in the regulation of hemoglobin and bicarbonate (HCO_3^-) involved in the acid/base balance of the organism [3]. It is important to explore and define the mechanisms that drive this unique cell to address wellness and chronic disease management [5].

2. Multiferroic influences on the erythrocyte's zeta potential

Upon examination of the red blood cell physiology, it is clear that both biochemical and electromagnetic influences may need to be defined and understood [6]. The lack of internal membranes and a nucleus in this cell shows it potentially operates very differently from most other eukaryotic cells. The plasma and internal membranes of other cell types are known to operate with a differential across the membranes, while the erythrocyte operates with the differential on the surface of this torus [7]. Therefore, the surface charge dynamics of the erythrocyte may be critical to its functionality. The red blood cell can be considered a type of *capacitor* in the organism due to the fact that the surface area on a capacitor is very important with regard to its function and efficiency [8]. A capacitor stores potential energy in an electric field with one or more pairs of conductors that are separated by an insulator or dielectric medium. A discussion of the proposed hypothesis of the process of how this unique cell may store energy through electric and magnetic (multiferroic) influences in the presence of a dielectric medium (chloride anion) in order to drive its zeta potential will now be presented.

The interaction of electric and magnetic orders in metal-organic configurations is known to exhibit more than one primary ferroic properties (multiferroic), that include ferromagnetism, ferroelectricity, and ferroelasticity [9–14]. Ferromagnetism occurs when a spontaneous magnetism is changed or switched by another applied field, ferroelectricity when a spontaneous electric polarization is switchable by an applied electromagnetic field, and ferroelasticity when a deformation that is switchable by applied stress occurs with all in the same phase [11]. Ferromagnetism is also considered a form of permanent magnetism (like that of magnets) where the time of decay of the magnetic field and its influence are reversed (time reversal) [15]. The presence of the ferromagnetic metal, iron, in the red blood cell speaks to a ferromagnetic influence that is present to reverse the time of decay of the magnetic field (time-reversal) of the erythrocyte [16]. Some scientists have believed iron only exists in the body as a weak paramagnetic ion, but this concept should be re-evaluated if this magnetization is switchable or time reversal symmetry may be occurring in the body due to a ferromagnetic influence.

Ferroelectric influences are known to exhibit a spontaneous electrical polarization that is switchable in an applied (magnetic) field [10, 17]. When we examine the surface of the toroidal erythrocyte, we see in order for the erythrocyte to function optimally, there needs to be a separation of the negative surface membrane charge from the positively charged Stern layer (cation layer). Chloride has been shown to modulate the voltage-gated chloride ion channels via its enhanced ferroelectric state under the influence of a DEP EMF [18, 19]. The diamagnetic chloride anion may also act as a dielectric constant to separate the charges (electrical polarity change in the presence of a magnetic field leading to breaks in spatial inversion symmetry or how particles orient in relation to each other or in space) on the membrane surface of the erythrocyte (negative surface membrane and positive Stern layer) to create static current flow and quite possibly an area for stored energy immediately surrounding the red blood cell (**Figure 1**) [15, 17].

This unique cell's membrane surface must maintain a static current surface membrane flow to remain free of other erythrocytes, cations, platelets, oxidative proteins, etc., in order for the optimal surface membrane exchange of oxygen (O_2) for carbon dioxide (CO_2) to occur in the body. In addition, Band 3/AE1 is an anion channel that appears to be gated by the diamagnetic chloride anion. If the cations in the plasma are interfering with or occupying the space at the negative membrane surface area, the Cl^- is not able to adequately surround the membrane in order to be readily available to conduct an exchange for HCO_3^- in order to maintain cell neutrality as it exits the cell as well as other possible intracellular functions that will be discussed.

Ferroelasticity is another ferroic property that we see in the *modus operandi* of the erythrocyte with regard to spontaneous strain, which can be seen in the deformability that is required of the red blood cells as they traverse the shear forces that

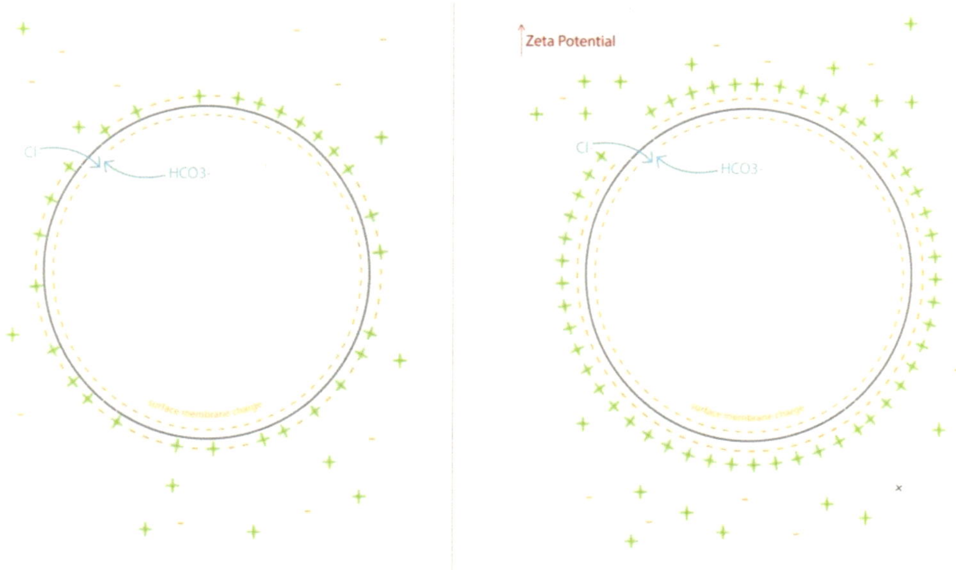

Figure 1.
Zeta potential of RBC. Decreased zeta potential is seen on the left with no separation of charges between the negative membrane surface and the Stern cation layer. Increased zeta potential on the right with separation of the negative surface membrane charge and the Stern cation layer (via ferroelectric change in chloride anion polarity).

exist in the vascular system. The shape memory effect can be seen as the erythrocyte deforms/flattens to traverse the smallest of capillaries in the microcirculation, without hemolysis (rupturing) to return to its previous biconcave discoid shape as it re-enters the circulation [20].

An interruption in the field driven by ferroelectric properties of chloride anion polarity (ferroelectric spatial inversion symmetry) and/or ferromagnetic properties of iron (ferromagnetic time reversal) may decrease or weaken the zeta potential. The zeta potential is a good measure of the electrical repulsive forces between particles as a function of distance. The zeta potential is also the critical control mechanism that offers stability of colloidal dispersions among the blood components [21]. The zeta potential (ζ) (Eq. (1)) equals the ionic strength (viscosity) of the medium (η), electronegative charge of the RBC membrane (electrophoretic mobility) (μ), divided by the dielectric constant (ε).

$$\zeta = 4\pi\eta\,(\mu)/(\varepsilon) \qquad (1)$$

The calculation of the zeta potential using the Smoluchowski equation (Eq. (2)) depicts electrophoretic mobility (μ) as equal to electric permittivity of the liquid (ε) divided by the viscosity (η) of the plasma (Eq. (2)). This is applicable when there is a thin double layer, stable zeta potential, with large colloidal particles (RBCs) and high ionic strength.

$$\mu = \varepsilon\xi/\eta \qquad (2)$$

Characteristic-based algorithms such as the zeta potential equation have limitations as they only govern measures in one spatial dimension in time where the direction of the phase velocity degenerates into an either positive or negative direction. We propose that the zeta potential (Eq. (1)) *also* requires an interaction between a break in time reversal (from ferromagnetic influence on serum iron) and spatial inversion symmetry (from ferroelectric influence in chloride) that maintains

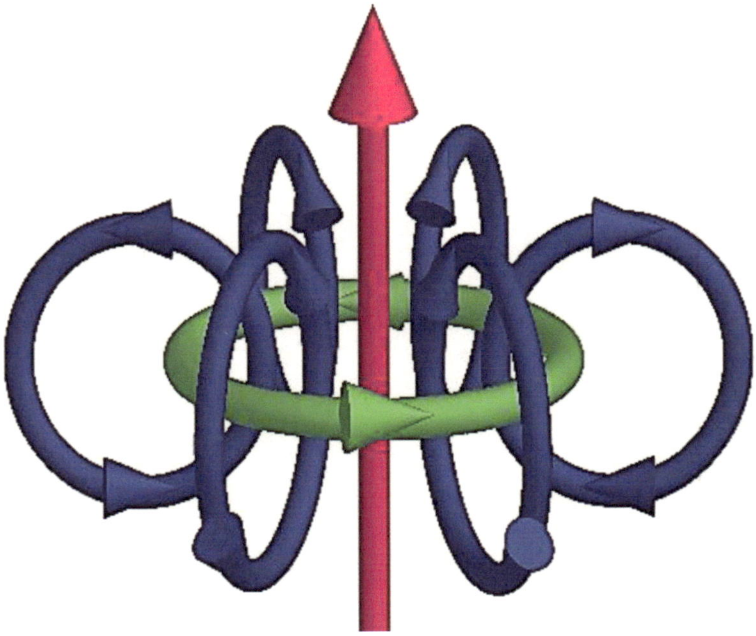

Figure 2.
Magnetic toroidal flow of the erythrocyte that may be fueled by the electrostatic field/zeta potential on the membrane surface. The green arrows represent the central separation chamber (pDEP and nDEP flow) with external separating forces being applied perpendicular to the flow (blue arrows) (Purnell et al. [3]).

separation of negative surface membrane area from the Stern layer (**Figure 2**). In order to add these measures to the zeta potential equation, multidimensional equations will be required to be split into multiple one-dimensional space-time formulations using both eigenvalues and eigenvectors.

The sign of the eigenvalue is an indicator of the direction of signal transmission, while the eigenvectors are the elements that are essential for diagonalizing the coefficient matrices. In the temporal-spatial planes, t-ξ, t-η, and t-ζ, eigenvalues are found by solving the sixth-degree characteristic equation that factors in the coefficient matrices [22]. It is also known that $\sigma = \sqrt{\mu/\varepsilon}$ contains the dimension of electric resistance. In space, it is commonly referred to as the impedance of lossless dielectric media [23]. Eigenvectors can explain the different coordinates (time points) of movements of a molecule at possible vectors and the eigenvalues can be used to describe the movement in and around the complex molecule [24]. Therefore, we hypothesize that the zeta potential may be most efficiently governed with consideration given to temporal-spatial changes that drive these multiferroic influences of ferromagnetism, ferroelectricity, and ferroelasticity that may be occurring in the red blood cell physiology.

2.1 Toroidal characteristics of the erythrocyte

It is known that an electric dipole consists of a pair of opposing charges and the magnetic dipole maintains a current loop [7]. The toroidal dipole is different because the currents flow on the surface of a torus. The red blood cell's unique design is a toroid where static currents need to flow on the surface of the torus in order to maintain efficient separation (possibly under the influence of the ferroelectric changes in the dielectric constant, chloride) of the positively charged Stern layer and the negative surface membrane charge [7]. This configuration of the external field is thought to be identically zero and the surface static currents create a magnetic field that is confined *within* the torus [7]. Therefore, this would lead to no interaction between the toroidal dipoles and the internal electric and magnetic fields [7].

The red blood cell may be viewed as exhibiting breaks in both ferroelectric (magnetic field driven, electric-spatial inversion symmetry) and ferromagnetic (magnetic-time reversal) influences that exhibit long-range order [25, 26]. Consequently, the red blood cell can be considered as a member of the toroidal multipole family since its physiology appears to require electric multipoles (red arrow) and magnetic multipoles (blue circles) that are driven by multiferroic influences (**Figure 2**). Theoretical works with toroidal resonances in natural media still remain in their infancy and tools to measure these phenomena are yet to be developed [27]. At the present time, re-examination of spectroscopic data/observations is warranted.

2.2 The Golden Ratio of the erythrocyte

The Golden Ratio is an irrational number, a function of phi, φ, and has been considered the most beautiful mathematical ratio in art, architecture, and nature for centuries [28–30]. The erythrocyte can be seen to display this Golden Ratio when one examines the size, shape, proportions, and curvature of this unique cell (**Figure 3**) [3].

The average diameter of the human red blood cell is 6.2–8.2 μm with the thickest point measuring 2–2.5 μm ($\sqrt{5}$) and the minimum thickness at the center of the toroid measures 0.8–1 μm divided by 2 for the two equal and opposing sides of the proportion to achieve 1.6803339887 (Golden Ratio of the red blood cell) (Eq. (3)).

$$\varphi = \frac{(1+\sqrt{5})}{2} = \mathbf{1.6180339887...} \tag{3}$$

The measurement of the center depth of the torus to the thickest point of the torus divided represents a measurable relative radial proportion of the Golden Ratio in the human erythrocyte. The normal and measurable range for the Golden Ratio would then be set into normal range values for the RBC (i.e., 1.4–1.75). It should be said that this ratio could be a notable biomarker that would require a lensless sensor imaging for point-of-care testing in order to disrupt the red blood cell's microenvironment as little as possible.

The microenvironment where this cell resides and maintains its multiferroic and field-driven component is critical to its function and for the maintenance of this Golden Ratio. Just as a snowflake is a water molecule that has frozen into its geometric proportions (Golden Ratio) falling/spinning through a specific microenvironment (freezing temperatures) within the field of the earth and must be examined before it is removed from these critical factors of formation, the red blood cell must be examined as close to its natural state (non-hemolyzed, non-anticoagulated, non-centrifuged etc.) in order to visualize its innate and natural state/physiology.

The maintenance of this Golden Ratio may have been underestimated since this living geometry of the red blood cell may be critical for efficient oxygen/carbon dioxide exchange as well as acid/base balance in the body [3]. The erythrocyte morphology and what guides this unique shape has been one of the least understood in the human body and it appears that biological shape and geometric changes are significant and can be linked to degenerative changes, embryogenesis, and even cancer [31].

2.3 Dielectrophoretic electromagnetic field flow fractionation in the Golden Ratio proportions of the erythrocyte

Since the geometric proportions of the Golden Ratio appear in nature, one must contemplate the significance of this geometry and why it occurs throughout nature. The Golden Ratio and its mathematically defined proportions of the erythrocyte

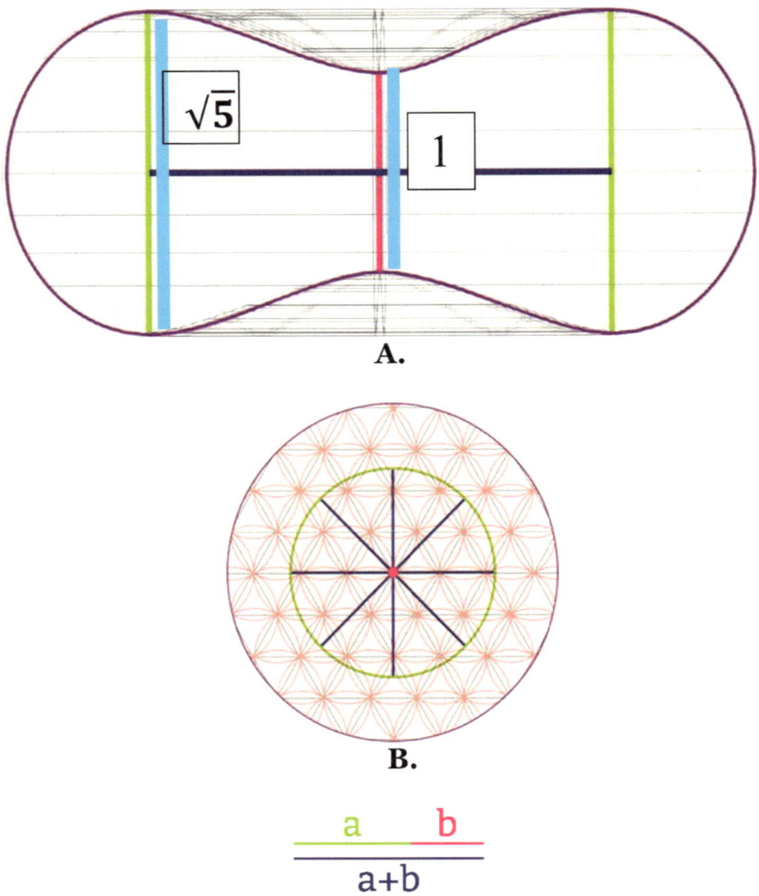

$$\frac{a+b}{a} = \frac{a}{b} = \varphi$$

Figure 3.
The Golden Ratio geometrical proportions of the erythrocyte. Upon cross-sectional analysis (A.), the sum of the quantities of the larger quantity (a + b) is equal to the ratio of the larger quantity (a) to the smaller one (b) and represents the entire Golden Ratio area of the erythrocyte or a measure of one representative radius (or measurable relative radial proportion) as denoted in Eq. 3. (B) The entire Golden Ratio area shown from top view of the Erythrocyte. The measurable relative radial proportion could be mathematically set into normal range values for the RBC Golden Ratio (i.e., 1.40-1.75) (Purnell, Butawan & Ramsey, 2018).

may actually house a dielectrophoretic electromagnetic field (DEP EMF), and these proportions may be critical for the proper physiological function of this unique cell. Recently, dielectrophoresis has been a topic of study due to its potential to manipulate microparticles and nanoparticles within and around cells [32]. Dielectrophoresis is seen to occur when a polarizable particle becomes suspended in a non-uniform alternating current (AC) or direct current (DC) electric field. This electric field polarizes the particle and if the particle moves in the direction of increasing electric field, then the behavior is positive dielectrophoretic (pDEP), and if the particle moves away from the high field regions, it is known as negative dielectrophoretic (nDEP).

According to the Maxwell-Wagner-Sillars polarization, this separation response occurs in conjunction with a necessary dielectric regulator or a field separator [33]. The concept of field separation through dielectric media has been well defined and understood in solid state electronics. It now appears the metal-organic applications in living organisms strongly speak to the need to apply and understand the field separation that may be necessary for membrane function in living things. Dr. Bruce

Lipton first offered the novel concept that the cell membrane is the cell's "brain" [34]. The membrane is a separator in the sense that it differentiates the cell from the outside world. There are mechanisms that control the membranes that have remained elusive to date. There appears to be a wisdom within cells and their membrane functionality that governs their behavior and physiology. The chloride anion may play a unique role in the gating of membranes through its dielectric properties and ferroelectric polarity changes it exhibits in and around cell membranes present in all cell types including the erythrocytes.

Just as the chloride anion is known to gate and modulate Band 3/AE1 on the surface of the erythrocyte torus, it may also play a role within the torus and especially within the area of the Golden Ratio that may serve as a dielectrophoretic electromagnetic field flow fractionation (DEP EMFFF) mechanism to process serum CO_2 (a cell respiration by-product within living organisms). We should note that water is a necessary component that is critical to both shield and amplify different charged species, serve as a high dielectric constant (ε), and is the known matrix of all living organisms [35, 36]. It is also known that water clusters may be able to transmit electromagnetic signals [37]. Therefore, water and CO_2 as H_2CO_3 (carbonic acid) are thought to enter the red blood cell from the plasma and can be seen as entering into a recycling arena within this unique cell. To date, carbonic anhydrase has been thought to be the enzymatic catalyst that separates H_2CO_3 into H^+ and HCO_3^- and is currently a topic of research across the globe [38–40].

We hypothesize that the negatively charged diamagnetic chloride anions and the static current they induce in and around the negative surface membrane charge and the Stern layer in the plasma (to drive zeta potential) may also drive the DEP EMFFF in the Golden Ratio of the proportions where the chloride anion continues to act as a field separator. This field separator action of the chloride anion and its ferroelectric changes in polarity within the magnetic field that resides within the Golden Ratio of the erythrocyte may fuel the DEP EMFFF in conjunction with the

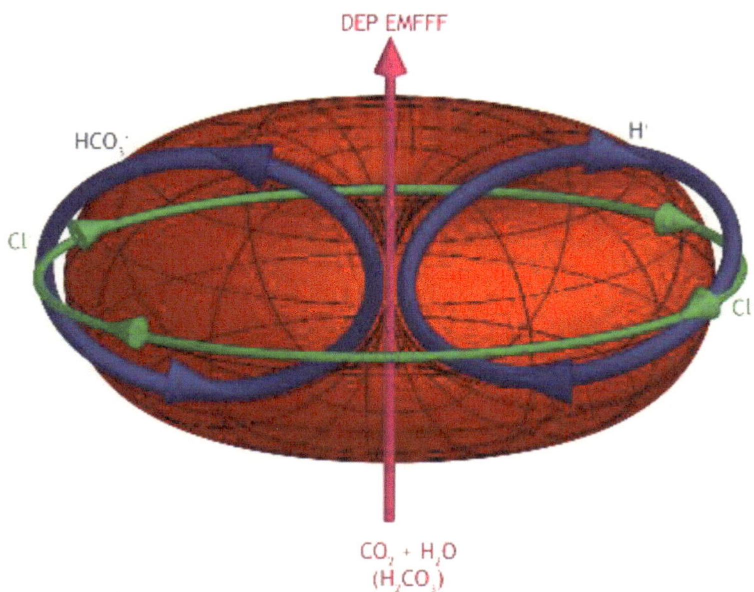

Figure 4.
Dielectrophoretic electromagnetic field flow fractionation of the erythrocyte. This DEP EMFFF, with the assistance of hydrodynamic (water) and dielectric chloride anion (Cl^-) influences, separates H_2CO_3 into positively charged H^+ (pDEP), which flows to the membrane surface (Hgb) to facilitate oxygen delivery and the negatively charged HCO_3^- (nDEP) exits into the plasma through Band 3/AE1 for acid/base homeostasis (Purnell et al. [3]).

hydrodynamic (dielectric influence of water) influences. The water and the chloride anion may induce a DEP separation of the positively charged H^+ (pDEP) which flows to the erythrocyte membrane surface to be used for hemoglobin function as the negatively charged HCO_3^- (nDEP) exits the cell into the plasma through the anion channel Band 3/AE1 for acid-base control in the body (**Figure 4**).

The chloride anion may again function as the separator of charge/flow at the red blood cell plasma membrane as the HCO_3^- (nDEP) is eluted from the cell and the chloride enters the cell to continue to its function within the cell. Parabolic velocity of the flow of these charged ions causes the HCO_3^- (nDEP) to move further away from the cell membrane in order to be eluted from the cell into the plasma as opposed to the H^+ (pDEP) that remains in the membrane for hemoglobin function [41]. The erythrocyte ideally recycles 70–75% of the serum CO_2 in the body (to H^+ and HCO_3^-) and generally only 20–25% of the serum CO_2 needs to remain available in the plasma for use by the lungs for regulation of acid/base homeostasis. The maintenance of the zeta potential and the Golden Ratio proportions may be a new area of future research for medicine and science [42].

3. Conclusion

The Golden Ratio proportions (possibly driven by the zeta potential) of the erythrocyte appear to offer clues to this cell's unique shape and function. Since biological shape and geometric changes can be linked to degenerative changes, it is important that we take notice of why and how these geometric shapes are important [43–55]. When there is a disruption in the zeta potential (toroidal surface) on the erythrocyte, this may lead to a loss of the Golden Ratio proportions (DEP EMFFF), geometric shape distortions, and decreased efficiency of CO_2 recycling as well as O_2 delivery with this most abundant and unique cell in our bodies [56].

Miniaturized lensless sensor imaging for microscopic visualization at point-of-care delivery is currently a research focus across the globe [57–59]. Due to the quantum microenvironmental factors that are critical to this possibly field-driven cell, it is important to examine these proportions with as little disruption to these factors as possible in order to quantify the Newtonian fluidics as well as calculations such as the Reynolds number. Future lensless imaging and examination of a newly drawn drop of blood may be the most valuable and accurate tool to evaluate the Golden Ratio along with the red blood cell's efficiency [47, 54, 57].

Conflict of interest

Marcy C. Purnell is the holder of "Biochloride Generation and Methods" International Application Number PCT/US18/14238.

Author details

Marcy C. Purnell* and Risa D. Ramsey
The Loewenberg College of Nursing, University of Memphis, Memphis, TN, USA

*Address all correspondence to: mpurnell@memphis.edu

References

[1] Diez-Silva M, Dao M, Han J, Lim CT, Suresh S. Shape and biomechanical characteristics of human red blood cells in health and disease. MRS Bulletin. 2010;**35**(5):382-388

[2] Pandy KB, Rizvi SI. Biomarkers of oxidative stress in red blood cells. Biomedical Papers. 2011;**155**(2):131-136. DOI: 10.5507/bp.2011.027

[3] Purnell M, Butawan M, Ramsey R. Bio-field array: A dielectrophoretic electromagnetic toroidal excitation to restore and maintain the golden ratio in human erythrocytes. Physiological Reports. 2018;**6**:11. DOI: 10.14814/phy2.13722

[4] Malmivuo J, Plonsey R. Bioelectromagnetism. New York: Oxford University Press; 1995. pp. 26-31. ISBN: 978-0195058239

[5] Du E, Dao M, Suresh S. Quantitative biomechanics of healthy and diseased red blood cells using dielectrophoresis in a microfluidic system. Extreme Mechanics Letters. 2014;**1**:35-42

[6] Purnell M, Whitt M. Bioelectrodynamics: A new patient care strategy for nursing, health and wellness. Holistic Nursing Practice. 2016;**30**(1):4-9

[7] Papasimakis N, Fedotov VA, Savinov TA, Raybould TA, Zheludev NI. Electromagnetic toroidal excitations in matter and free space. Nature Materials. 2016;**15**:263-271

[8] Ho J, Jow RT, Boggs S. Historical introduction to capacitor technology. IEEE Electrical Insulation Magazine. 2010;**26**(1):20-25

[9] Fiebig M, Lottermoser D, Frohlich A, Goltsev V, Pisarev RV. Observation of coupled magnetic and electric domains. Nature. 2002;**419**:818-820

[10] Kimura T, Goto T, Shintani K, Ishizaka K, Arima T, Tokura Y. Magnetic control of ferroelectric polarization. Nature. 2003;**426**:55-58

[11] Hur N, Park S, Sharma PA, Ahn JS, Guha S, Cheong SW. Electric polarization reversal and memory in a multiferroic material induced by magnetic fields. Nature. 2004;**429**(6990):392-395

[12] Cheong SW, Mostovoy M. Multiferroics: A magnetic twist for ferroelectricity. Nature Materials. 2007;**6**:13-20

[13] Tian Y, Stroppa A, Chai Y, Wang S, Barone P, Picozzi S, et al. Cross coupling between electric and magnetic orders in a multiferroic metal-organic framework. Scientific Reports. 2014;**4**:6062. DOI: 10.1038/srep06062

[14] Qi W, Xu B, Ren S. An organic approach for nanostructured multiferroics. Nanoscale. 2015;**7**(20): 9122-9132

[15] Eerenstein W, Mathur ND, Scott JF. Multiferroic and magnetoelectric materials. Nature. 2006;**442**:759-765

[16] Chikazumi S. Physics of Ferromagnetism. 2nd ed. Oxford: Oxford University Press; 2012. ISBN: 9780199564811

[17] Basu T, Adroja DT, Kolb F, Krug von Nidda HA, Ruff A, Hemmida M, et al. Complex nature of magnetic field induced ferroelectricity in $GdCrTiO_5$. Physical Review B. 2017;**96**:184431

[18] Purnell M, Skrinjar T. The dielectrophoretic disassociation of chloride ions and the influence on diamagnetic anisotropy in cell membranes. Discovery Medicine. 2016;**22**(122):257-273

[19] Purnell M. Bio-electric field enhancement: The influence on hyaluronan mediated motility receptors in human breast carcinoma. Discovery Medicine. 2017;**23**(127):259-267

[20] Chien S. Red cell deformability and its relevance to blood flow. Annual Review of Physiology. 1987;**49**:177-192. DOI: 10.1146annurev.ph.49.030187.001141

[21] Kirby BJ, Hasselbrink EF. Zeta potential of microfluidic substrates: 1. Theory, experimental techniques, and effects on separations. Electrophoresis. 2004;**25**(2):187-202

[22] Shang J. Computational Electromagnetic Aerodynamics. Hoboken, New Jersey: John Wiley & Sons; 2016

[23] Kraus JD. Electromagnetics (Electrical and Electronic Engineering). New York: McGraw Hill; 1953. ISBN 978-0070353954

[24] Sneha P, Doss CGP. Molecular dynamics: New frontier in personalized medicine. Advances in Protein Chemistry and Structural Biology. 2016;**102**:181-224

[25] Ederer C, Spaldin NA. Towards a microscopic theory of toroidal moments in bulk periodic crystals. Physical Review B. 2007;**76**:214404

[26] Spaldin NA, Fiebig M. The renaissance of magnetoelectric multiferroics. Science. 2005;**309**(5733):391-392

[27] Raybould TA, Fedotov VA, Papasimakis N, Kuprov I, Youngs IJ, Chen WT, et al. Toroidal circular dichroism. Physics Review B. 2016;**94**:035119

[28] Zhang XJ, Ou-Yang ZC. The mechanism behind beauty: Golden ratio appears in red blood cell shape; 2016; arXiv: 1608.01637v1 [physics.bio-ph]

[29] Abu-Taieh E. An algorithm for human modeling in information technology multimedia using human biometrics found in golden ratio, vitruvian man and neufert. In: Fifth International Conference on e-Learning, Manama, Bahrain; 2015. DOI: 10.1109/ECONF.2015.43

[30] Livio M. The Golden Ratio: The Story of Phi, the World's Most Astonishing Number. New York: Broadway Books; 2008

[31] Levin M. Reprogramming cells and tissue patterning via bioelectrical pathways: Molecular mechanisms and biomedical opportunities. Wiley Interdisciplinary Reviews: Systems Biology and Medicine. 2013;**5**:657-676. DOI: 10.1002/wsbm.1236

[32] Kirby BJ. Micro- and Nanoscale Fluid Mechanics: Transport in Microfluidic Devices. New York: Cambridge University Press; 2010. ISBN 978-0-521-11903-0

[33] Kremer F, Schönhals A. Broadband Dielectric Spectroscopy. Berlin Heidelberg: Springer-Verlag; 2003. ISBN 978-3-540-43407-8

[34] Lipton BH. The Biology of Belief. Carlsbad, CA: Hay House Inc.; 2008

[35] Kurian P, Capolupo A, Craddock TJA, Vitiello G. Water-mediated correlations in DNA-enzyme interactions. [physics.bio-ph] arXiv: 1608.08097; 2017

[36] Pollack GH, Figueroa X, Zhao Q. Molecules, water and radiant energy: New clues for the origin of life. International Journal of Molecular Sciences. 2009;**10**(4):1419-1429

[37] Montagnier L, Aissa J, Ferris S, Montagnier JL, Lavallee C. Electromagnetic signals are produced by aqueous nanostructures derived from bacterial DNA sequences. Interdisciplinary Sciences. 2009;**1**:81-90

[38] Wind TC, Messenger MP, Thompson D, Selby PJ, Banks RE. Measuring carbonic anhydrase IX as a hypoxia biomarker: Differences in concentrations in serum and plasma using commercial enzyme-linked immunosorbent assay due to influences of metal ions. Annals of Clinical Biochemistry. 2011;**48**(2):112-120

[39] Vince JW, Carlsson U, Reithmeier RA. Localization of the Cl^-/HCO_3^- anion exchanger binding site to the amino terminal region of carbonic anhydrase II. Biochemistry. 2000;**39**(44):13344-13349

[40] Wieth JO, Andersen OS, Brahm J, Bjerrum PJ, Borders CL. Chloride-bicarbonate exchange in red blood cells: Physiology of transport and chemical modification binding sites. Philosophical Transactions of the Royal Society of London. Series B, Biological Sciences. 1982;**299**(1097):383-399

[41] Davis JM, Giddings JC. Feasibility study of dielectrical field-flow fractionation. Journal of Separation Science and Technology. 2006;**21**(9):969-989. DOI: 10.1080/01496398608058390

[42] Rice M, Ismail B, Pillow MT. Approach to metabolic acidosis in the emergency department. Emergency Medicine Clinics of North America. 2014;**32**:403-420

[43] Ertan NZ, Bozfakioglu S, Ugurel E, Sinan M, Yalcin O. Alterations of erythrocyte rheology and cellular susceptibility in end stage renal disease: Effects of peritoneal dialysis. PLoS One. 2017;**12**(2):e0171371

[44] Serroukh Y, Djebara S, Lelubre C, Boudjeltia KZ, Biston P, Piagnerelli M. Alterations of the erythrocyte membrane during sepsis. Critical Care Research and Practice. 2012. 7pp. DOI: 10.1155/2012/702956 8/23/17

[45] Bai G, Li Y, Chu HK, Wang K, Tau Q, Xiong J, et al. Characterization of biomechanical properties of cells through dielectrophoresis based cell stretching and actin cytoskeleton modeling. Biomedical Engineering Online. 2017;**16**:41. DOI: 10.1186/s12938-017-0329-8

[46] Kim J, Lee HY, Shin S. Advances in the measurement of red blood cell deformability: A brief review. Journal of Cellular Biotechnology. 2015;**1**(1):63-79

[47] Giovanna T. Biomechanical properties of red blood cells in health and disease towards microfluidics. Biomicrofluidics. 2014;**8**(5):051501

[48] Hierso R, Waltz X, Mora P, Romana M, Lemonne N, Connes P, et al. Effects of oxidative stress on red blood cell rheology in sickle cell patients. British Journal of Haematology. 2014;**166**:601-606

[49] Babu N, Singh M. Influence of hyperglycemia on aggregation, deformability and shape parameters of erythrocytes. Clinical Hemorheology and Microcirculation. 2004;**31**(4):273-280

[50] Ahmad S, El-Sayed MS. The effects of graded resistance exercise on platelet aggregation and activation. Medicine and Science in Sports and Exercise. 2003;**35**(6):1026-1032

[51] Baskurt OK, Meiselman HJ. Blood rheology and hemodynamics. Seminars in Thrombosis and Hemostasis. 2003;**25**(5):435-450. The Hyperviscosity Syndromes. Thieme Medical Publishers: New York, NY

[52] Piagnerelli M, Zouaoui Boudjeltia K, Vanhaeverbeek M, Vincent JL. Red blood cell rheology in sepsis. Intensive Care Medicine. 2003;**29**:1052-1061

[53] McHedlishvili G, Maeda N. Blood flow structure related to red cell flow:

Determinant of blood fluidity in narrow microvessels. The Japanese Journal of Physiology. 2001;**51**(1):19-30

[54] Wang C, Popel A. Effect of red blood cell shape on oxygen transport in capillaries. Mathematical Biosciences. 1993;**116**(1):89-110

[55] Hung TC, Pham S, Steed DL, Webster MW, Butler DB. Alterations in erythrocyte rheology in patients with severe peripheral vascular disease: 1. Cell volume dependence of erythrocyte rigidity. Angiology. 1991;**42**(3):210-217

[56] Qiang Y, Liu J, Du E. Dielectrophoresis testing of nonlinear viscoelastic behaviors of human red blood cells. Micromachines. 2018;**9**:21. DOI: 10.3390/mi9010021

[57] Liao SH, Chang CY, Chang HC. A capillary dielectrophoretic chip for real-time blood cell separation from a drop of whole blood. Biomicrofluidics. 2013;7(2):024110

[58] Rauf A. A dielectric study on human blood and plasma. International Journal of Science, Environment and Technology. 2013;**2**(6):1396-1400

[59] Gurkan UA, Moon S, Geckil H, Xu F, Wang S, Lu TJ, et al. Miniaturized lensless imaging systems for cell and microorganism visualization in point-of-care testing. Biotechnology. 2011;**6**:138-149. DOI: 10.1002/biot.201000627